How I Became A Nurse Entrepreneur

Tales from
50 Nurses in Business

National Nurses in Business Association

Library of Congress catalog number: 91-90235

ISBN: 1-888315-03-2

Design and Production Coordination by **Revolution Designs**

Printed in the United States

Published by :
Power Publications
56 McArthur Avenue
Staten Island, NY 10312
1-800-331-6534

987654321

Table of Contents

Chapter 1

The Sky's the Limit

by Laura Gasparis Vonfrolio, RN, PhD, CEN, CCRN

Dependent—too dependent. I used to breathe, eat, and sleep my job—and I do mean job—at the hospital. Giving, giving, giving; constant approval-seeking behavior, aiming to please, whether it be patients, head nurses, or supervisors. You name it, and I was out to please it. Dependent on my job for my salary, feeling comfortable with the security of having a full-time job. One day it hit me. This is nauseating!

I also thought about the fact that I was working sixty hours a week as a staff nurse. I was working like a dog! And for what? Personal satisfaction? Huh! That's a joke. How do you get satisfaction when you are so busy that you're unable to do anything the way it should be done. Oh, I did the best I could. But down deep I knew that even doing the best I could, given the undesirable working conditions, I was not giving the best care the patient should have.

I verbalized, I gave my nursing leaders (who by the way, perpetuated this horrendous environment) suggestions and feedback. But I quickly learned if you don't sing the same tune as the male-dominated bureaucratic institution, stay mute. For I have learned that within a hospital setting, having a mind, a mouth, and a brain—and heaven forbid, using all three of these at the same time—could get you labeled as a troublemaker. Once in a while all three would manifest themselves and uh-oh, there I was being counseled for my "bad atti-tude." Then it hit me. Where am I, Russia? Nursery school? Who are these people? My parents? What the hell is happening to my brain? Enough!

I was blaming my circumstances for my mental apathy and life's boredom. I decided to take charge of myself. I decided to rid that self-immobilizing unhappiness in myself. Although I was not re-gretting what I had done, it was what I hadn't done that was torment-ing me.

I came home and announced to my roommate that I was going to start a business and asked her if she would like to join me. "A busi-ness, what the heck do we know about a business? What would we sell? What do we have in common?" she asked.

"CPR," I responded. "We will sell CPR!"

She said, "Who is going to buy CPR, the Red Cross and The Ameri-can Heart Association do it for free don't they?"

"If you put a price on something, people will buy it, nobody wants something for free," I responded. "I'll find someone to buy it." (*Lesson: Make up your mind to do something about your ideas.*)

So I typed two letters. "Dear Employers: We are two registered nurses who will train your employees in a life-saving skill known as CPR..." I went on to tell them how important CPR training is, that when a bystander is certified in CPR it may save lives, and who knows, it may save your very own life! I sent out only two letters. One to Merrill Lynch and one to E.F. Hutton.

Two weeks later, the phone rang. "Hello, this is Merrill."

Merrill, I thought—who the heck would name their kid Merrill?

"Merrill who?" I asked.

"Merrill Lynch," the woman responded.

I turned to my roommate and asked her, "Lisa, do you know a Merrill Lynch?"

"Merrill Lynch, you jerk, didn't you send them a letter?"

"Oh yeah," I responded.

The woman asked, "Is this CPR Associates?"

"Yes, CPR Associates, that's who we are." I was glad she said that, as I had forgotten what I called my company in the letter I had sent out two weeks ago!

She went on to say that she had approximately 540 employees to train in CPR. Wow! 540 people. Quite a bind I got myself into, as I didn't even have an updated CPR card, let alone a business in it. I told her that we were very busy and that we would have to get back to her with some dates.

I hung up the phone and was just ready to go into shock, when the phone rang again. "Hello, CPR Associates, how may we help you?"

"Hi, this is Mr. Stern from E.F. Hutton, and we have 560 employees to be trained in CPR."

"Well, Mr. Stern," I replied, "we are very busy now, may I take your number and call you when we have openings?" (*Lesson: Act, think, and talk with conviction at all times.*)

I hung up the phone and collapsed. I was in a panic! I was not even currently certified in basic CPR, let alone certified to be a CPR *in-*

structor. Off to the hospital I went to work. I finally got a CPR card and then enrolled in a CPR Instructor course. I went to the bank and took out a $10,000 loan. I took out a personal loan (I lied and told the bank that I had lost 150 pounds and needed to buy a new wardrobe), and then bought ten mannequins.

I placed an ad in the newspaper for CPR instructors. I received about twenty-five applicants and chose ten to work for my new company. I called E.F. Hutton and Merrill Lynch and arranged to teach their employees. We taught approximately 100 employees in the morning and 100 employees in the afternoon, as we were teaching a four-hour Heartsaver course.

Would you believe that in the midst of all this commotion I forgot to think about what I was going to charge? I remember, when asked by the head of the Personnel Department what the fee per person was, I stated $20 a head.

He hit his hand on the desk and repeated, "Twenty dollars a person!"

 I immediately replied, "How about $15 a person?"

He said, "OK that's fine, the last time we had a CPR course they charged us $60 a person."

Boy, did I goof! (*Lesson: Keep your mouth shut until all the cards are on the table.*)

Well, upon completion of the first two accounts, I came home Friday night with two checks totaling $16,000. Not bad for a week's work! I paid my instructors very well, paid off the bank loan and had $2,000 for myself.

I decided then to go full blast with this business. (*Lesson: Get big results by believing big.*) I sent a mailing out to small and large companies exhorting the importance of CPR training— "...and the life saved may be your very own." The calls came in. *(Lesson: Always count your chickens before they hatch!)* Doctors' offices, dentists' offices, health clubs, nursery schools, daycare centers, mothers, PTA's (I guess no sense doing lunch duty if you don't know what to do when a kid chokes), busdrivers, lifeguards, aerobic instructors, schools, restaurants; it was endless. *(Lesson: The sky's the limit.)*

We decided to also offer CPR parties. It's like a Tupperware party, only instead of demonstrating Tupperware, we demonstrate CPR in the comfort of one's home. They get a group of ten or more people together, and we will show up with manequins and teach them in their own home. Upon completion of the course, we give the family a sticker to place on their front door. It's like the "in" thing to have! We also have monthly CPR courses held at a local hotel for the community. *(Lesson: Use your mind for thinking and dreaming, not simply as a warehouse for facts.)*

We presently educate approximately 3,000 people a year and will be looking to offer CPR training outside of New York. *(Lesson: Think progress, believe in progress, push for progress.)*

Believe it can be done. When you believe something can be done, your mind will find the ways to do it. Believing a solution paves the way to solution. Think success, don't think failure. Thinking success conditions your mind to create plans that produce success. Thinking failure does the exact opposite. Failure thinking conditions the mind to think other thoughts that produce failure.

Believe *Big.* The size of your success is determined by the size of your belief. Think little goals and expect little achievements; think big goals and win big success. Remember that ideas alone won't bring success. Ideas have value only when you act upon them. Elevate your cerebral machinery to the point where you act out of choice—your choice.

The trick to being an entrepreneur is to gamble your time, not your money.

Don't think that you are wandering into a business alone. There is plenty of help out there. The banks want to help you. Your family and friends will certainly want to help you. You will even find that Uncle Sam has some lovely tax advantages for you. You will also discover that you have inner resources that you don't know about until you push yourself beyond some of your traditional limits.

Believe in yourself fully, for no activity is beyond your potential. Open yourself up to new experiences, for boredom is debilitating and psychologically unhealthy.

Laura Gasparis Vonfrolio, RN, PhD, CEN, CCRN
President, Education Enterprises
President, Power Publications
President, National Nurses in Business Association
Publisher, REVOLUTION—The Journal of Nurse Empowerment
56 McArthur Ave.
Staten Island, NY 10312
1-800-331-6534

Chapter 2

Nurse Entrepreneur...
What Are You Waiting for?

Laura Gasparis Vonfrolio, RN, PhD, CEN, CCRN

As an owner of four businesses related to nursing, I have been up many nights, thinking, not about my businesses but... *"Why don't nurses market their services? Why aren't there more nurse entrepreneurs? Why doesn't academia offer a nurse entrepreneurship course as an elective in their masters program?"*

Here we are a multi-talented, very intellectual, organized, dedicated group of individuals who have a very marketable service—nursing service—yet most nurses rely on a weekly paycheck for those services they render for an institution that sometimes creates an environment in which we are unable to do our best. (Ouch...the truth may be painful!)

The answer to the question why nurses don't market their services could take up a whole book! But my purpose in this article is to excite you and to explore the possibilities for nurse entrepreneurship. Please be assured that I am not advocating that nurses leave the bedside or hospital setting, for you can still practice and be a nurse entrepreneur. Having a successful business does wonders for you mentally & physically. It increases your self-esteem as well as your bank account!

INDEPENDENT PRACTITIONERS

As best stated by Helen Borel (1992), "My fellow American registered nurses, what are you waiting for? All of you are already licensed to be self-employed as independent practitioners!" I never understood (and I guess neither does Helen) why nurses don't form corporations and market their nursing services back to the hospitals or to those individuals needing orthopaedic nursing in the home setting.

For nurses to band together and form corporations and market their services to hospitals is an idea for the future. For now, we can get our feet wet in the entrepreneurial sense and market orthopaedic nursing service to patients in the home setting. The home market for your nursing service could include:
* Trauma patients sent home in traction and or with external fixators
* Patients with total hip/total knee replacement
* Children with developmental and congenital problems such as spinabifida, cerebral palsy, muscular dystrophy, arthogryposis, osteogenesis, imperfecta, congenital dislocated hips
* Outpatient management of Lyme disease and Osteomyelitis

Now let's briefly go through the steps of starting a home health care business. In order to become a provider for nursing care in the home setting, you will need to identify the carrier for Medicare that has jurisdiction in your location and your state Medicaid agency. Research the market for third party payment sources such as HMOs, Blue Cross/Blue Shield, etc. Write to the payers requesting information and an application to become a provider to their beneficiaries. It is advisable that you see an attorney to incorporate your business and inquire about insurance as there can be liability with this type of service business. A good resource for the nurse interested in third party reimbursement is *A Sourcebook For Healthcare Providers* written by Motta and Whitaker (1992) and published by GK Publications, 2210 N. Illinois Street, Belleville, IL 62221.

CASE MANAGEMENT

Organizations such as insurance companies, corporations and industries are increasingly utilizing third party reviewers to evaluate case management. Currently, most third party reviewers are independently contracting their services to businesses. Nurse-owned case management companies would coordinate, oversee and manage the care so that it is cost effective for the insurance company, corporation or industry seeking your service. A nurse-owned company called Quality Review Associates provides education seminars to prepare nurses for this career opportunity. They are located at 11818 Gateway Blvd., Los Angeles, California 90064.

PUBLISH

How about putting together a review book for the NAON certification examination. It's easy! All you need is a vision (book with your name on it) and determination. Send a letter to 200 clinical nurse specialists in orthopaedic nursing asking them to submit 5-10 questions with answer rationales. You can buy hospital lists from any list broker found in the telephone directory. I usually use MMS list brokers in Chicago. Ask them to print the name and address of the hospital with Attention: Orthopaedic Clinical Nurse Specialist. From my experience with writing review books (eight to date) you will probably get questions from approximately 50 nurses. This will give you anywhere from 250-500 questions. Analyze them, research the answer rationales, check the references and Voila! A Book!

You now have to make a decision. Either publish it yourself or submit it to a publishing company. If you send it to a publishing company submit a table of contents, one or two chapters and a prospectus. A prospectus sells your manuscript to the publishing company. It explains why your book is needed, how it is better than the competition, and who your market is for such a book. The publishing company may offer you anywhere from 8%-15% royalty per book. The other option is publishing the book yourself. There are lots of printers in the United States who print books; just check your yellow pages. I use BookMasters in Ashland, Ohio for printing my books, as they have a quick turnaround and are relatively inexpensive. Give them a call at 1-800-537-6727 and ask for information. A three hundred page book, 6 X 9 in size usually runs around $2.00-$3.00 per book. If you sell your book for $15.00, that's a nice profit for you! An excellent resource for self-publishing is *The Self Publishing Manual* by Dan Poynter, published by Para Publishing in Santa Barbara, California, 1-800-PARAPUB.

SEMINARS

Put yourself on a brochure! Yes, market your expertise! If you keep your price low and your topics broad you can get an audience. Orthopaedic nurses have lots of information that ER, critical care, medical-surgical and home care nurses would love to know!
There are two ways of marketing yourself as a consultant:
1. Direct mail key people in the hospitals who will utilize your services for their staff as you would provide an onsite seminar for their nurses.
2. Rent a hotel conference room, direct mail to your potential audience, and offer your seminars.

The best way (unless you have written several books, articles, or are very well know to all) is to market yourself on a brochure and entice individuals to attend your seminar. In this way you will then be approached by attendees to do an in-house consultation/presentation. Also on your brochure you can advertise that you are available for on-site presentations, which saves the hospital money rather than send its nurses out to seminars.

So let's go through the steps of marketing yourself on a brochure.

SIX MONTHS BEFORE PROJECTED PROGRAM:

1. Get A Name!

Register your name as a business with your county clerk's office. Set up a bank account in the business name. Give yourself a name that is broad in scope such as Seminars Unlimited, Nursing Education Associates, Educational Affiliates, National Nurses Network, etc. There are some drawbacks for using your own name. People usually don't like writing out a check to a person. Individuals think that it's more credible writing it out to a company. You don't have to incorporate this business; just get yourself business papers. Call your county clerk's office and they will tell you what is needed. It is usually just a matter of filling out three forms and costing you around $35.00!

2. Get An Act!

For a full day program you will need 4 one hour and fifteen minute presentations. Make sure to include a lot of areas/objectives in a presentation description on your brochure. The more on the brochure the better the course is perceived by the attendees. Don't limit or narrow your topic so that content goes into picayune little things. For instance, don't have a course entitled, "Orthopaedic Emergencies in Patients with Renal Failure".

3. Get Course Approved for CEUs!

Contact the appropriate accrediting body for guidelines. You can contact your state nurses' association or specialty associations. Follow them to a TEE. Once you get approval you will be able to buy a mailing list from the accrediting organization. Accreditors usually want: Program Description, participant objective, content outline, bibliography, schedule of presentation, post-test. The fee for approval usually costs anywhere from $25.00- $85.00 and is good for one-two years.

4. Get A Location!

Try to put a few locations on one brochure to increase cost effectiveness. Cluster the locations, so that you can target your mailing list.

Make them in cities in the same state, but too far from each other to drive. If you are going to go to different states, schedule them in one section of the United States.

5. Get a Hotel!
Contact hotels and arrange for conference rooms. Wait for contracts from hotels before printing your brochure. Call around! Big differences in prices. Bargain, wheel and deal. They do decrease their prices when provoked. Usually booking a seminar 15 minutes outside of a big city location can cut costs by 75%.

6. Get Bulk Rate Permit!
Go to the post office and obtain a bulk rate permit. Make sure this permit number is on your brochure. Minimal cost, about $60-$75 yearly. Enables you to mail out at .16 -.19 cents a brochure as opposed to .32 cents (Saves you $100 per 1000 brochures).

FIVE MONTHS BEFORE PROJECTED PROGRAM
7. Get A Brochure Together!
This can be done by the printer, or you may want to consult with a graphic artist. When created...Read and re-read your brochure proof over and over. There are always mistakes that you don't see if you just look it over once. Have your friends read it, have your mother, father, husband, significant other read it! Anybody! REMEMBER: Format of brochure needs to be concise, easy to read.

8. Get A Printer!
Make sure you price around! Big differences in prices! You will have to make decisions regarding the kind of paper, the size of paper, ink color, folding. I have used Econocolor-Ohio Valley Post Litho in Florence, Kentucky. They not only print my brochures but mail them out too. Give Mike Stewart a call at 1-800-877-7405 for information and prices. I saved over $100,000.00 in printing expenses the first year that I used them!

FOUR MONTHS BEFORE PROJECTED PROGRAM
9. Get Mailing Lists!
Decide whether you want pressure labels or cheshire. You can order these from the accrediting body that issued you CEUs or from nursing journals. Remember that 100 brochures mailed usually gives you one to three responses. Send direct mail to nurses *and* hospitals, for only 1/4 of nurses subscribe to journals.

10. Get A Mailing House!
A mailing house will put the labels of names and addresses that you purchased and affix them to the brochures, sort and bulk according to the postal regulations and deliver them to the post office for mailing. Some printers will do mailing and some don't. You can find a mailing house in the yellow pages under..... "Mailing House!" The usual cost is around $20.00 per thousand brochures.

VIDEOS FOR PATIENTS
How about making a video for patients who are being discharged from the hospital or those patients seeing an orthopaedic physician for a specific disorder? This video would improve the patient's outcome and healing time, or would make acceptance and/or adjustment to the disorder easier. Patient education is the key for healthy healing. You could market these videos directly to physicians' offices or to patient education departments in hospitals. Or how about a video about orthopaedic nursing and sell it to nursing schools. Gee, what a great idea! If I had time I would make up a whole series; critical care nursing, labor & delivery nursing, oncology nursing, etc. What a nice package. I'm sure nursing schools would be interested. Get started now!

I hope that I have sparked an interest in entrepreneurship. Please believe in yourself fully, for no activity is beyond your potential. Open yourself up to new experiences, for boredom is debilitating and psychologically unhealthy. Believe it can be done. When you believe something can be done, your mind will find the ways to do it.

13

Think success; don't think failure. Thinking success conditions your mind to create plans that produce success. Thinking failure does the exact opposite. Failure-thinking conditions the mind to think other thoughts that produce failure. Believe BIG. The size of your success is determined by the size of your belief. Think little goals and expect little achievements, Think big goals and win big success. Remember that ideas alone won't bring success. Ideas have value only when you act upon them. Elevate your cerebral machinery to the point where you act out of choice....your choice.

Lastly, don't think that you are wandering into a business alone. There is plenty of help out there. Your family and friends will certainly want to help you. You may even contact me for guidance and support. I can be reached at 56 McArthur Avenue, Staten Island, New York 10312, 1-800-331-6534. You will even find that Uncle Sam has some lovely tax advantages for you. You will also discover that you have inner resources that you don't know about until you push yourself beyond some of your traditional limits. Go for it!

References

Borel, H. (1992). Powerquake in Nursing. *REVOLUTION - The Journal of Nurse Empowerment,* Winter, 36-42.

Motta, G. & Whitaker, K. (1992) *Reimbursement: A Sourcebook for Healthcare Providers.* Belleville, IL.:GK Publications.

Poynter, D. (1991) *The Self Publishing Manual.* 6th ed. Santa Barbara, CA: Para Publishing.

Vogel, G. Doleyah, N. (1988) *Entrepreneuring: A Nurses' Guide to Starting a Business.* New York: National League of Nursing.

Chapter 3

The Nursing Cycle of Success

by Carolyn S. Zagury, MS, RN

(This updated profile first appeared in the Winter, 1994 issue of *REVO-LUTION — The Journal of Nurse Empowerment*)

I would never have predicted that two years after founding my first company, Professional Healthcare Associates, Inc. (an education and consulting firm) in 1989, I would also own Vista Publishing, Inc. and, in 1996, become Vice President for development of a home health care company. Although I had always thought about starting my own business, I could not imagine that I would have the skills or talent to be an independent businesswoman! Now —all these years later—I actually have three businesses!

Even after more than 18 years in various nursing practice settings and management positions, I was naive enough to believe that nurses could make a difference from within organized healthcare, especially in a senior management position. So when the hospital in which I worked gave me the title of Assistant Vice President for Strategic Services, I thought it a wonderful opportunity for change. After all, this was a large teaching hospital, progressive, forward thinking, etc. The nurses, physicians and allied health professionals with whom I worked were anxious for change, to be progressive and to make a difference.

The problems we encountered centered around an administration that did not want change—"business as usual" was the norm. For nearly three years the battles raged until, finally, a physician colleague helped me focus on the problem, telling me that I was "not their kind of team player and, if I was to survive, I would have to see things their way."

After a lot of soul searching my decision was clear. I could not, and would not, compromise my values and beliefs. With the full support and understanding of my husband, David, I resigned and the first exciting journey— Professional Healthcare Associates, Inc.—began.

Many things have changed at PHA since 1989. I am now the sole owner of the company and services have been streamlined to meet the needs of every client. These services include strategic planning for nursing, geriatric service development, grant writing and teaching nursing programs across the country.

Educational programs are tailored to meet individual needs and focus on business skills for nurses, management issues and empowerment. Examples of teaching topics include "The Business Side of Nursing Management," "The Human Side of Power and Influence," "Writing for Publication," "Making A Difference: The Nursing Cycle of Success," and "Nurse Entrepreneurship: Building Toward the Future."

While teaching nursing programs, I met nurses from all around the country and many asked me about publishing. They were not as concerned about clinical manuscripts, but rather creative works such as poetry, biographies, fiction and non-fiction. Since a colleague and I had just completed a nursing leadership training manual and we were about to look for a publisher, the timing was right to explore the world of publishing.

I called hundreds of publishers! Small ones, large ones, every size imaginable. The answers were the same: "What would a nurse know about writing!" "There is no market for nurses." "We don't need any more women in the fiction markets, especially nurses." "Nurses should push bedpans not pens." "We don't need a Danielle Steele with a cap on." Almost 100% of these responses were followed by laughter! I was outraged! Surely someone would recognize the talent in our profession. But, no one did!

My research also revealed that approximately 400,000 manuscripts are submitted to publishers each year for possible publication. Of these, less than 10% are targeted for promotion. The responses I had received about nurse-authors clearly did not leave me with much opportunity; publishers were interested in larger, more traditional clinical textbooks. Not the creative side of nurses.

My choices became clear. Either forget about pursuing this any further or accept the challenge and do something about it! The end result—Vista Publishing, Inc. was begun in March of 1991.

I knew very little about the publishing business and was really starting from the ground up. After reading as many books, newsletters, and articles as I could, I spoke with my friend and mentor, Laura Gasparis Vonfrolio at A.D. Von Publishers. I learned about ISBN numbers, the Library of Congress Catalog Numbering System, Writer's Market, Books in Advance, wholesalers, distributors, and copyright submissions, among other things. With all of this information in hand, I sought the advice of an attorney and an accountant to establish Vista Publishing, Inc.

The primary goals of Vista are to provide an alternative forum for nurse and allied health professional authors to promote books with a positive image of nursing and health care. An image that will celebrate the "whole" person—beyond the clinical excellence for which nurses are so well known. There is no stronger communication tool than the written word! I believe that 2.2 million nurses have much to celebrate, individually and collectively, and a tremendous amount of power to make a difference!

A challenge that was originally fueled by anger has now become a challenge that is charged by excitement and discovery. The authors who are part of the Vista family are incredible people; 95% of our authors are nurses who come from every area of nursing—from the bedside to research and education, and even one who works with the United Nations on international issues of disaster and mass trauma. In early 1997, our first physician-authored medical mystery will be published! The talent and creativity in our profession is remarkable! Perhaps the most significant quality I have found is that nurses write with an honest and straight-from-the-heart approach, the same way they approach their professional practices.

Vista Publishing is classified as a small press. We currently have 36 titles in print with a fully committed publishing schedule into mid-1999, with more manuscripts arriving each week. Most of our authors come through referrals and inquires.

Publishing a book is a long process and may take from 18-24 months to be in print. Each step is time consuming and human-resource intensive. The author, editor, publisher and graphic artist work together to maintain the momentum and the excitement of the finished product.

Marketing for a small press presents many challenges. It is difficult to get books into bookstores since most deal through wholesalers and distributors. Vista has been very fortunate to have been accepted by several large firms. However, we still deal through specific small press programs that order based on customer demand. Other marketing strategies include direct mail to customers, nursing schools, libraries, as well as radio talk shows for author interviews and book signings at local bookstores by the authors. We also exhibit at nursing conferences and work with other exhibitors who act as distributors.

Each author is very active in the marketing of her/his book and since our authors are from all over the country, including Alaska, it is essential that they participate in arranging local book signings, interviews and actual sales.

Another very important marketing tool is book reviews. We look for as many avenues for book reviews as possible through the news media and nursing journals. An on-going goal for Vista is to convince nursing journals that book reviews for non-clinical books are appropriate and that a "non-traditional" book honors the "whole person." The parts of a nurse cannot be separated into professional and "other"—the total person is the nurse!

Vista has been lucky to have so many nurses believe in our goals and offer to help in "spreading the word." For those interested in promoting our books, we offer a sales sub-contract and pay a small commission. This avenue has been effective in terms of networking and getting our name into the marketplace.

A very special marketing tool is networking with other nurse entrepreneurs. For those of you who choose to own your own business, you will find that other nurse-business owners are your strongest supporters. Sharing the marketplace and helping to promote each other's products and services seems to be a natural for nurses! Laura Gasparis Vonfrolio has been not only an inspiration, but one of the strongest supporters of Vista Publishing. Many other nurse entrepreneurs have also encouraged and supported Vista products.

As PHA and Vista Publishing, Inc. continued to grow and to foster opportunities for nursing, I began to feel strongly that I would like a challenge that would focus more on clinical issues. I was actually beginning to miss the clinical interventions. I was fortunate to meet Helen Vaughn, BSN, RNC, the President and Founder of ElderHome Care, Inc., a proprietary home care agency. We had many discussions about advancing the business. These meetings provided us the opportunity to get to know each other and feel comfortable working together. Our goals and our love of geriatric nursing are very similar.

Now, in 1997, I have again taken on a new challenge of working in the home care field. It is truly exciting and rewarding. The work load has indeed tripled, but this is a consequence of business ownership that I welcome. It is another journey toward making a difference for my profession!

Exploring the world of nurse entrepreneurship is an open opportunity, especially in today's changing healthcare environment. Never before have nurses had so many professional alternatives available to them.

I am sure that you will find, just as I have, that fellow nurse entrepreneurs are your most important asset and the link to the world of hard work, long hours, independence, commitment, fun and a financially secure future.

Professional Healthcare Associates, Inc.
Vista Publishing, Inc.
ElderHome Care, Inc.
473 Broadway
Long Branch, NJ 07740
(908) 229-6500   Fax: (908) 229-9647

Vista Publishing, Inc.
A Nurse Owned Company

Below is a sampling of the titles available through Vista Publishing, Inc.
For a complete list of books available, call **1-800-634-2498**.

Cast Into the Fire
by Carolyn Chambers Clark, EdD, RN

A novel based on historical fact and set in the great fabled era of witch hunts. In an age of political corruption, **great deeds and mighty people survive.** Follow Ventura and her family across two continents as they struggle with the evils of the 17th century Seville and Salem. *Ventura sweeps into history when she learns the power of the wise woman and dares to be a healer.*
Price: $14.95

Medicine Bow
by Beth Roberts Kotarski, MSN, CRNP

A powerful novel based on historical fact that will take the reader on a long and courageous journey with Rachel Dunham, RN. The story begins in New York City in 1879. Through a twist of fate, Rachel travels to Medicine Bow, Wyoming to accept a challenging nursing position. A position that tests not only her abilities as a nurse, but her strength as a woman. *Rachel's courage will make us all proud to be a nurse and...proud to be a woman!*
Price: $14.95

Signs of Life, Observations of Death
by Craig Betson, RN, MHA

An extraordinary collection of poetry that allows the reader to join Craig in sharing the intense emotions that nurses feel in the situations they face every day. You will enter their world. You will learn what drives them to be, and what makes them work with such compassion and strength.
Price: $9.95

Murmurs
by Carol Battaglia, RN, BSN

A wonderful and inspirational collection of original poetry and essays. Each poem and essay encourages the reader to reach beyond our self imposed boundaries and... *"hear the murmurs of life."*
Price: $12.95

Not Old, Not Full of Days
by Norma Singer, RN

A powerful and moving novel about nurses, friendship and commitment. Learn the extraordinary lessons of friendship. Learn to treasure the power of friendship!
Price: $16.95

To Be a Nurse
by Linda Strangio, RN, MA, CCRN

An eloquent collection of short stories that portray the love of the author for her profession and for the patients that she has cared for. Join Linda in tears, laughter and caring. Each story will bring the reader a very personal glimpse of the real meaning of nursing and the special people who have chosen the finest of all helping professions. Discover what it means **TO BE A NURSE!**
Price: $12.95

Nurse Entrepreneur:
Building the Bridge of Opportunity
by Carolyn S. Zagury, MS, RN, CPC

This comprehensive book/workbook will help the aspiring nurse business owner to explore their abilities, determination and commitment to enter the exciting and challenging world of business ownership. Chapters by an accountant and an attorney will help to focus on the start-up requirements and commitments of owning a business.
Price: $21.95

Health Assessment: Spanish/English Version
by Diana V. Sanchez, RN, BSN

A must read assessment book for nurses in all clinical settings who work with Spanish speaking clients. A comprehensive, easy to understand manual, written in Spanish and English that will guide the nurse system by system through the client assessment.
Price: $24.95

Nurturing the Nurse on the Path to Success
by Carolyn Travis Laskey, RN

An excellent guide for nurses who aspire to climb the ladder of success. You will need to stretch and take risks. This book will help to build self esteem, identify growth opportunities and expand expertise...*the basic tools for self empowerment...Nursing's mandate for the 1990's!*
Price: $16.95

Protect Your ASSets:
The Nurses Self Defense Guide
by Audrey Stephan, EdD, RN

Become **"A Winning Bedside Warrior!"** Learn the factors and situations of malpractice and how to work through the many elements of fear if named in a suit. The author's strong background and "front line" experience make this book a must read for all nurses!
Price: $12.95

Chapter 4

A Daughter's Perspective: My Mom

by Valerie Gray RN, MS

Let me take a few minutes of your time to tell you about my mom— super mom, nurse entrepreneur, and a rather nice lady.

When I was just a wee tyke of seven (1976), she launched her first business venture amidst my crayons and finger paints. Her memos and phone messages (we shared an office—our family room and my playroom) were frequently splattered by my paints, but she never minded. I was well trained to answer the phone and ask politely, "Who's calling please?" I was frequently mistaken for an older four-teen-year old despite my seven-year-old voice.

This business venture involved organizing seminars aboard cruise ships from the Port of Miami, Florida, for nurses, physicians, and other healthcare workers. My best friend and I had no complaints. We accompanied my mom on seven cruises in two years to twenty-five different ports. We learned about behavioral objectives, slide projectors, handouts, registration blanks, seminar evaluations, con-tracting for speakers, continuing education units, and most impor-tantly, to direct the participants to where the restrooms were.

After two years of suffering through twelve "sea" seminars and nu-merous "land" seminars, Mom shifted gears. Shucks, I had just gotten my CPR down pat and was sure that at the age of nine, I could save anyone's life if the occasion arose. We taught over 3,000 people in all aspects of emergency and critical care and made a few pennies along the way.

Her next venture was with her nurse friend. They became experts in medical malpractice and the litigation on this subject. This venture was a puzzlement to me, now a twelve-year old. I found the cute guys on the cruise ship much more interesting than the lengthy telephone calls and long analytical reports put together for self-insured and insurance companies detailing liability, standard of care, proximate cause, and teaching folks how to act during a deposition.

However, I was advised that she had become an advocate for an injured patient and that were few brave advocates in 1982 for "malpracticed" patients, especially nurses. This business venture grew from one portable tape recorder to three computers (which luckily had Pac Man), a national list of clients, and lots of great trips for me to Chicago, San Francisco, New York, and Boston to accompany Mom while consulting.

She stayed active in this business until March 30, 1983. I remember this date because I was in a very serious accident. A coma ensued for three months (of course, I don't remember), but God, my mother, and some great Intensive Care Unit nurses snatched me from the jaws of death. After four months in the hospital, Mom brought me home. The business had closed—no way she could keep it up and be with me eighteen hours a day. I never asked, but she was just there every day—all day.

We came home and it was a difficult two years. I wasn't supposed to have lived. There wasn't a facility for a fourteen-year old head-injured, middle-class gal like me, so Mom became my rehabilitation and catastrophic case manager. She knew nothing of rehabilitation— she always told me it was too boring and that she didn't like it. But as the next few years passed, I noted that she had a new specialty.

People called and asked her advice on physical therapy, cognitive rehabilitation, good speech therapists, and appropriate programs for brain injury. She later became a vocational counselor, too. So, of course, Mom had a new venture. I think she liked this one—she could really help people who had nowhere else to turn. *Case Manager* is what she was now. I had just learned to describe litigation to my friends, and now I had to explain case manager. Some friends thought that Mom worked in a large warehouse and was in charge of large cases of goods. Those folks required a lot of explanation.

This venture grew from five files/clients to more than 100 in two years, a part-time secretary in the spare bedroom next to my room to a suite of offices, five clerical people, and four other nurses. She was really organized with this one. She knew about Sub-S corporations, capital expenses, independent contractors, Federal I.D. Numbers, profit and loss statements, staff meetings, employee development, and marketing.

I, of course, had graduated from high school and started college and was called upon frequently to assist Mom, visit some of the patients with her, and give my overall input. My crayons had been exchanged for highlighters, data entry terminals, and collating copy machines.

Mom is revered by her nurse friends who remember her when they all worked in the county emergency room, saving lives eight hours a day—blood, guts and gore, they called it. She now wears executive clothes to work every day (with some guidance from me, as I have great taste in clothing).

By financial standards she's doing very well, doubling the gross revenues of this business each year to the present. She really did it for me. She wanted a flexible schedule to enjoy being a mom. She attended my school functions without permission from a boss, drove

25

me wherever I needed to go, and did not have the pressure of a work schedule arranged by another.

She's very conscientious and rather compulsive, so she always does a good job. All her accounts like her, and so, of course, business prospered. She learned how to do all this rehabilitation from taking care of me, and she's an expert in brain injury. I guess you could say Mom learned during these past twelve years that she's become an entrepreneur. She always told me to be ethical, don't compromise your values (in the long run you'll prevail), organize, prioritize, network, never be afraid to ask, trust your instincts, and treat people like you wish to be treated. Very simple rules not specific to a nurse, but all she ever really followed—and it worked for her.I guess you could say her job description of Rehabilitation Specialist served her well, too. She had to rehabilitate herself. I left Mom in 1987. God let me stay with her for four years, five months and fourteen days (she's the one who did the counting) after my accident. Now, I am part of her life from that place they call Heaven. I'm not disabled here, and for that I'm sure she's glad, but I know she'd rather have me with her.

That's my mom, the nurse entrepreneur who has succeeded in the case management business. I love her, and I know she loves me.

UPDATE 1997

You met Valerie Gray through me, her daughter Kimberly. I have been asked to give you an update regarding Valerie Gray's business activities since her story first appeared in 1991 in *How I Became a Nurse Entrepreneur.*

My mother, Valerie Gray, has continued to grow her business in leaps and bounds since 1991.

She took on a very bold move and relocated herself that year to New England. From that location, she continued to operate, long distance, her business in the Southeast area, covering Florida, Georgia and Alabama, as well as developing new business in the New England area. In spite of her ignorance of computer technology, she utilized modems, e-mail, facsimiles, beepers and overnight delivery to accomplish this task. Of course now in 1997, it is pretty common practice and everyone is doing the same thing, including delving into the internet.

She also felt a burning need to acknowledge me, her daughter, and in 1992, began yet another business, that of her avocation and passion. Horses. My mother and her husband now operate a large, recreational horseback riding academy in Southern Vermont that includes Bed and Breakfast accommodations, trail riding, a full horseback riding academy, including English, Western and Dressage disciplines of riding, wagon rides, sleigh rides and pony rides. She basically practices what she preaches in her vocational activities with her clients, that of utilizing your avocation to turn them into a profitable business.

She still travels to Florida frequently to oversee that operation. She also travels extensively around New England to oversee the New England operation; as well as travel around the U.S. for other consultations.

It has now been nearly a decade that she has lived life without her daughter. It never gets easier. She has just learned to deal with it. If you travel to Vermont, you will see that the farm is named "Kimberly Farms." Guess why?

Valerie Gray, RN, MS
Valerie Gray Case Management
P.O. Box 350218
Ft. Lauderdale, FL 33335
(305) 462-4470

Chapter 5

Nurse-Publisher Finds Her Niche

(This profile appeared in the January 1990 issue of the *Nurse-Entrepreneur's Exchange.*)

Editor's Note: **Attention Nurses**, *founded in 1985 by Michelle Lowder, RN, is a bimonthly publication mailed free to 150,000 nurses, hospitals, agencies and nurse-related companies in Southern California.* **Attention Nurses** *advertises employment opportunities, continuing education programs, and other services of interest to nurses, such as nursing associations, uniform shops and nurse-to-nurse businesses.*

NEE: Tell us about your nursing background.
Michelle: "I graduated from nursing school in 1981 and right away went into critical care, specifically respiratory intensive care. Then I went to med/surg ICU, and then into neuro ICU. I dabbled in pediatrics, and then in a weight loss clinic—I couldn't find my niche."

*NEE: How did you conceive the idea for **Attention Nurses**?*
Michelle: "I had a transition job with a medical equipment company in a non-sales capacity, but because of my RN, I was making a lot of sales for them—sales that I was not getting compensated for. They didn't see the rationale behind hiring me as a nurse in a higher posi-

tion in sales, so we parted ways, and I started looking for another job in medical sales.

During that period I saw a need for a resource for continuing education originally. I knew the classes my hospital offered, I saw what came in the mail, but I also knew there were a lot of other CE programs out there. I thought it would be a good idea if there was a one-stop publication for available CE programs in Southern California— so I bought a mailing list and some art supplies, got some advertising clients, and started."

NEE: Where did you obtain the publishing skills required to produce **Attention Nurses**?
Michelle: "I had taken a graphic arts class in high school which was very interesting to me from a creative point of view. In terms of being artistic, I can barely write my own name—but I have good ideas. In graphic arts you have to do things freehand. In high school I also worked in the business office and learned basic accounting, which has helped a lot in my own business."

NEE: Did you use computers and desktop publishing software when you started in 1985?
Michelle: "No. Desktop publishing was just starting back then, so I began in the traditional way. Since it had been a long time since high school, I hired a graphic artist to do the pasteup.

About a year later desktop publishing came into its own, so I bought a Macintosh computer and later a laser printer. I have recently hired another person who also does typesetting, so we now have two computers."

NEE: Advertisers are the main source of revenue for **Attention Nurses**. *How did you originally approach them?*
Michelle: I just got on the phone, and presented them with a logical, less-expensive means of reaching the largest number of nurses. So

I'd call and say, "This is it—do you want it? It's a good idea, how about it?" I figured it was a numbers game—the more people I called, the more advertisers I'd get. We started off mailing to 45,000 nurses, and over time expanded county by county. In January, 1987, we expanded to Los Angeles county, and that's when it really took off. We're now mailing to 150,000 nurses.

We actually started out with two separate publications. One version went to two counties, and the other version went to a different county. We did that because we thought people in Orange county would not be interested in advertising to people in Palm Springs. After nine months,we decided it was easier for everyone, the advertisers and myself, to do just one publication for everybody."

*NEE: How has **Attention Nurses** grown in size since its inception?*
Michelle: "My first issue was two pages,8 1/2" x 11." We are now up to twenty-four pages, and growing from there. We are reaching more nurses than any other publication in Southern California."

NEE: What's been your greatest challenge?
Michelle: "Doing everything myself that has to be done with your own business—being the sales person,the boss,doing the bookkeeping, learning the computer, emptying the trash!

Now I'm to the point where I have some employees and don't have to do everything. I have a sales person and an assistant who does the accounting, helps put the marketing package together, and helps the sales person generate advertisers."

NEE: What has been your greatest satisfaction?
Michelle: "Being the boss! It's double-edged, because the responsibility of being the boss is that if you screw up, there's no one else to go to. The nice thing is that if I have a good idea, I can make it happen—if you're working for someone else, that isn't necessarily

the case. It's not that I have trouble with authority, it's just that I have good ideas.

The feedback I get from nurses is great! I receive letters saying how much they appreciate *Attention Nurses* as a unique recourse. They like it because it has different kinds of things than the newspapers; for example, there's a lot of unusual job opportunities advertised.

One difference between *Attention Nurses* and other nursing publications is that nurses read it for the ads. Since there are no articles, they are not distracted. People placing ads in other publications hope that a nurse reading it will also happen to see their ad. The focus of *Attention Nurses* is that nurses look at it to find the advertisers."

NEE: Any tips for nurses starting a business?
Michelle: "Know something about the business you are starting. I had some graphic arts skills, and I had a few business skills.

My father was self-employed, so I knew what it was like to not get a regular paycheck. I would advise nurses to remember that you may not make nursing wages the first couple of years. Try to keep everything in the business you can, and take just enough to live on.

Try to be proactive instead of reactive. Don't put your head in the sand when you see a problem. Attack it with vigor!"

Attention Nurses
249 N. Brand Blvd., Suite 308
Glendale,CA 91203
(818)972-2701

Chapter 6

Marketing Approach to the Nursing Crisis

by Richard C. Thompson, RN, PC

On August 28, 1988, our third child and first son was born to my wife and I. Amid our joy, I mentioned to my wife that I would not return to work until after the Christmas holiday as to facilitate bonding for all of us and to enjoy the birth of our last child.

What occurred over the next four months, however, was not planned.

I had been working in a combined twelve-bed medical-surgical intensive care unit since 1984. At this time, to complement our home situation related to in-home child care, I was working every Thursday, Friday and Saturday night, 7 p.m. to 7 a.m. In addition to this, I had sought extra shifts through a national agency in other ICU's while my wife remained on maternity leave.

While working five to six nights a week for three months or more, I had become quite disillusioned with my future as a nurse, since I felt I was killing myself with a minimal return. I had been toying with the idea of going back to school for an MBA since business had always interested me. The turning point was when I inadvertently discovered what this agency had been charging for my services;it was then I realized that I was being paid less than 50 percent of the fee. Needless to say, I was quite miffed.

33

At this point I decided to enroll at a local state college in pursuit of an MBA. One of the first courses I enrolled in was marketing, which I enjoyed very much. The final paper was to be a case history of a company and its potential for changing its present marketing approach. Many different ideas were evident in relation to simple changes that could be implemented in any hospital that would, in return, make staff turnover a thing of the past as well as make staff morale soar.

The more I thought of it, the more realistic the idea had become. Most hospital administration-employee relations are based on 19th century thought to begin with. This is certainly not the path on which to implement reform. With the nursing situation in its present demise, why not give nurses the option to choose their own situations, minus benefits, and a pay scale second to none?

I presented this to my professor prior to my research and asked him if I could utilize this concept rather than presenting a company that would have no interest in such a radical change. He agreed and gave me his blessings.

My intent was also to test the waters in order to see if it actually was a viable concept in practice, not just on paper. I approached two hospitals with the idea of cutting out the middle-men, who in this case were the agencies. During my employment with agencies, it had gotten to the point where the hospitals were calling me directly, or I was calling them for time. The only task the agency was performing at this time was handling the money—and keeping a large part of it to boot! Their first response was one of disbelief. "How could you even imagine to propose such a thing?" "It can't possibly be legal in New York state to do that." "You're way ahead of your time." (I think you get the picture of what I was up against.)

Talking with my wife over breakfast the next day, I said I had no idea how to approach this concept. I had already scanned the computer at the hospital where I was presently employed, looking for journal articles related to independent contracting. There were none—worse yet—the only reference available was related to measures that could be taken to *prevent* nursing administrators from utilizing supplemental nursing services. All at once it hit me; I had worked at the Rochester Public Library during high school and remembered that in the General Reference section there was a large selection of Yellow Pages from all over the country. What if I looked under the *Nursing* heading and sought out single names? Surely these people would be independent!

I rushed downtown and began to pore over the books. Within two hours I had compiled a list of twelve names from all over the country, including Boston, Chicago, Atlanta, and Houston. As soon as I arrived home, I began to call the numbers on the list. The first eight numbers were dead ends. The next call was to a nurse in Boston who was attempting to bring nurses from Great Britain to work in her area. She was independent and working as a consultant to nursing homes. This conversation really picked up my spirits, proving to me that a nurse does not have to be employed by an institution to function as a nurse.

The last call was to a nurse in Houston, and lo and behold she was an independent contracting critical care nurse! I could not believe it. She have me the number of the organization that placed her, and I called immediately. We spoke at length about my idea and how I thought it might be implemented. He was astonished that I had never heard of it already functioning in the Southeastern United States. My case history proceeded with this information.

If I could do backflips, I would have been doing them at this point. I called the New York State Department of Education to check for any statutes against a staff nurse offering services as an independent contractor; the person stated that to her knowledge there weren't, but why would I want to do something like that anyway? I said, "If I could help the image, professionalism, and compensation of the critical care nurse, why not?" She did not have a response to that.

Living in New York all my life, and knowing how tough regulations can be, I decided that if New York state would incorporate me as a professional, it would alleviate any questions of legal status and thus quell a hospital's fears. This procedure succeeded very nicely.

In the meantime, I had received my case history, titled "A Marketing Approach to the Nursing Crisis" back from my professor. That same night he called me at home wanting to talk about my paper. For the next fifteen minutes he did all the talking, and I was in awe. He could not believe that the nursing profession had been allowed to progress to its current state. He went on to say that all other professional occupations have opened up for women and asked, "Why would young people subject themselves to this sort of mistreatment?" He thought my idea was outstanding and that I should consider offering my paper for publication.

I was floored. I had no idea that someone else, let alone someone outside the profession, would give my presentation such high marks. After my acute cerebral swelling decreased, he encouraged me to follow through with it and give it my all—which I did.

In the state of New York, a registry is an employment agency for professionals licensed and regulated by the New York Department of Labor. A nursing agency is just that; the nurses are their employees. They are regulated by the Labor Department and Department of Health. To add to this confusion, it takes six to twelve months to obtain a registry license and one to four years to obtain an agency license.

My philosophy in my business is to give the nurse using the Registry's placement service a majority of the fee charged to any institution, which to this day I do. To my knowledge, these nurses are the highest paid outside of New York City. The means by which the quality of nurses is maintained at a high level is simple; I don't advertise. Nurses are aware of the Registry by word-of-mouth, and thus far the quality of nurses has been very high.

After becoming incorporated, I again approached the two hospitals with a formal agreement and proposal for their review. Uncertain of the time frame required to formalize contracts with the two hospitals, I applied for, and was offered, a nursing supervisor position at a 363-bed skilled nursing facility in the Rochester area. The Director of Nursing at the SNF was completely understanding of my situation and asked me to take four or five days to think about this impending change in my life.

As I mentioned to my wife when I arrived home, there was nothing to think about. The starting pay was more than I was presently making, and the atmosphere was much more relaxed. I decided, however, to wait the five days prior to notifying them of my decision.

On the morning of the fifth day, I was cutting the lawn when my wife called me in to take a phone call. It was one of the two hospitals I had approached, and the administrator wanted to know if I was still interested in contracting my services. I was elated! Within seven days I had thanked the director at the SNF for the opportunity of employment and declined the position. On the seventh day I met with the hospital administrator, who promptly signed the agreement; I was to start the next night.

As I walked from the hospital to the car, I had never felt in so much control of my own destiny prior to this moment, and I truly believed that this was only the beginning! I had, with one swoop of the pen, doubled my income working four hours less a week. As I look back now, there would have been no way I could have afforded the start-up costs of my business on my previous salary; being independent not only made it affordable but comfortable.

I had been reading many books on industry, including a few by Tom Peters and Buck Rogers. The most important messages I found were simple: give the best service available, set the highest standards for the people you place, and don't pull punches with the institutions who use your service. I have done this consistently, and I base this on comments from the hospitals who are very impressed with the professionalism and dependability of the nurses using the Registry's placement services. The hospitals are guaranteed that if I agree to cover a shift, and the nurse cannot fulfill her end, I will personally cover it myself. In the first year I have had to turn down no more than six shifts.

In the March 1990 issue of the *American Journal of Nursing*, there appeared an article entitled, "Agency Nurse vs. the IRS: Are You an Employee, an Independent Contractor, or Both?" by Sally Sumner, RN; Pam Grau, RN; and attorney Barry Frank, Esq. I called and spoke with Sally that afternoon and was quite surprised to learn of the IRS tactics affecting our industry. I was equally surprised and excited to learn of Sally and Pam's success over the past eight years in placing independent contractors in critical care units.

I slowly began to learn that there are many registries across the country who are placing nurses in the same fashion. I attended a workshop on independent contracting at the 1990 ANA conference in Boston and was impressed with the turnout and the opportunity to meet with other people in the same business.

I also attended the NNBA conference in Washington, D.C. in November of 1990, and following informal conversations with many of the same people who were in Boston, we formed a network. Those in attendance agreed to start a national organization that will focus our opposition to IRS tactics against independent contractors. This has grown out of a strong belief that nurses are professionals and should be recognized as having the choice to be independent in an ever-changing marketplace.

The past two years have been exciting and challenging for me. It seems that perhaps I got into nursing to leave a viable impression on an industry whose time has come.

The ball is in our court now. Do we run with it or give it back to the powers that have created the present crisis in the American health system? We are the movers and the shakers of the 21st century, and there is no time like the present. We *can* make a difference.

UPDATE 1997

To state that there has been some change to our industry since this book was first published would be an understatement.

Managed Care, Preferred Providers, the nursing glut, new RN's unable to find work other than working as aides, hospital consolidation, Patient Care Techs, Home Health Aides—the list goes on and on.

The most staggering reality of today's healthcare industry is that the patient is not the primary focus anymore—the bottom line is. This is totally evident in our hospitals today—understaffed and barely any nurses in sight. Paraprofessionals is the buzz word today—multitalented at a fraction of the cost. Clean room, pass trays and then give patient care is a scary reality today. Bottom line? It's more cost effective.

Let's move to home care. New York State, in their infinite wisdom, has developed a new care matrix for Home Health Aides. Some of the tasks that are to be allowed are the following: obtaining a blood glucose via a glucometer, taking the reading, documenting it and injecting insulin. Trach suctioning, NG and foley irrigation and sterile dressing changes. I have and will continue to refuse to place Home Health Aides into these situations. Of course, all the training must be absorbed by the employer, and the liability is yours as well. It is quite obvious to me that the whole rationale behind this is to save money. Period. To hell with the patient, the nurse and their professional license and the agency's license as well. You may correctly assume that all liability is on the supervising nurses' license. Not only are the situations unsafe and unprofessional, it is also unethical. I feel it is pretty poor for anyone to assume that a non professional with nothing to lose can operate under a professional's license who has everything to lose. Boy, you do not see too many doctors and lawyers running for the same concept in their professions now, do you?

Now that I have that off my chest, things here in Rochester, New York are just wonderful! I no longer operate my independent contractor Nurses Registry. I now own an employee based staffing and home care company. Five years ago I sold my soul to become part of a national organization, which funds my payroll and provides billing and back room support. My operating company, Flower City Health Care Services, teaches Frank Poliafico's (from Emergency and Safety Programs, Inc.) Smart CPR and Bystander Care with very good success. We have also provided risk management consulting services in the past.

Looking back, it's been one helluva ride—rollercoaster that is. Anyone in business knows that one minute you're on top of the world and the next you could be drowning. Looking forward, the proverbial rug is being shook out as you read this—the mom and pop organizations are going to have a tough go at it. My alliance with a national company has certainly helped, yet the major contracts on a national basis are very low in profit margin. I have discovered that you must niche—find it and expand it. Do not go overboard—too many avenues will overwhelm you. But on the other hand, don't keep all your eggs in one basket. The loss of a major contract could send you into a tailspin.

It used to be said that the healthcare industry changes rapidly—month to month. Today it seems it is hour to hour. We are keeping our general focus, yet remaining flexible enough to turn on a dime. The past eight years has been a priceless education, and hopefully the next eight years will be as fruitful.

Flower City Health Care Services
Village Gate
274 N. Goodman Street Suite A 302
Rochester, NY 14607
716-244-3362

Chapter 7

Entrepreneurship: Passion, Belief, Perseverance

by Mary Jones, RN, MN

Before I begin my saga which will explain my passage into the world of entrepreneurism, I would like to share something.

I personally had no inclination towards starting my own business. I was frustrated with my own current working situation, but I realized that no job was perfect. Almost every nurse shares a certain amount of frustration about the current state of the nursing profession, so I just looked at the good parts of my position and lived one day at a time.

In 1982, I began working as a nurse practitioner for a large OB-GYN group consisting of five gynecologists, one midwife, and myself. There were rumors that they were planning to hire a second midwife. It was beginning to look and feel more like a dynasty. It seems as if everyone in this community knew this medical practice.

My responsibilities included non-stress testing on the prenatal patients who required this and seeing patients who had scheduled appointments to specifically see me. Another part of my job included teaching prenatal classes which were equally divided into a class for each trimester. My master's degree was in Obstetrical Nursing, and I loved to teach, so this part of my job was interesting and fun. I was allowed to create the classes, including the format and handouts, and the classes were very well attended.

As I continued to teach the same set of classes over and over, the challenge of keeping them interesting for me increased. My personality, though, is one that loves challenge, so I kept reading the literature, changing the handouts, altering my jokes, and trying different techniques to generate enthusiasm. Little did I know that each Thursday while I was teaching I was being observed by a perinatologist who came up from Pasadena to do ultrasounds and amniocenteses. I always enjoyed Mark because the patients loved him, he had a great sense of humor, and his interests were diverse. One day out of the blue, he asked me why I was continuing to work for someone when I had such an ability to reach the patients. I had no idea what he was talking about, but I did start to listen. Slowly the idea began to crystallize, but the stumbling block was that he was challenging one of my greatest assumptions: a nurse practitioner had to work for a physician. Well, *didn't she*?

I continued to feel flattered by Mark's faith in my abilities, but I didn't have any plans to leave my comfortable nest. Well, as fate would have it, I went to a seminar on PMS. I had become active in the PMS movement and participated actively at the seminar because I had so many feelings and ideas about PMS. I believed that we were approaching it from the wrong perspective, and I wanted to generate some new thoughts from the participants. This was during the time PMS was just being recognized here in the United States, and there was so much controversy swirling around. After the seminar I was approached by several physicians and asked where my practice was located. They were very surprised to learn that I was in an OB-GYN office working for a group. One physician finally said,"Why don't you open your own practice and test your theories?" When I began to hear the same data from a variety of sources I started to actively pursue the possibility.

Now I was facing the ultimate challenge. Where does one begin? There was no National Nurses in Business Association in 1985. There were no nurse practitioners in independent practice in Ventura County. There were very few nurses anywhere who were doing what I wanted to. I began to search, and finally found a nurse practitioner who was in private practice, and who was willing to share with me. The focus of her practice was on women's health but concentrated on the areas of birth control, annual exams and abortions. I knew that I did not want to include abortions as part of my focus. My visualization was to develop a practice that would include education for women, a resource center, and a safe place where they could explore options regarding their own levels of wellness. I wanted to continue to provide gynecological exams, so I knew I would need a physical backup. I also discovered a yen for public speaking and decided to incorporate seminars into my visualization. So now that I had the dream, where would I start?

I began speaking with friends and my husband. The idea was a fascinating one, but was it realistic? Other questions kept coming up: Why would I leave a safe haven for the unknown? Why would anyone want to see me when they could see a real doctor? Why should a physician in the community help me anyway? Since Mark had started this whole process, I went back to him with my list of questions, and we began to solve each one. It had never occurred to me that my dream would not work, so I just viewed each adversity as a challenge. First, I found an attorney with a caustic wit but a great legal sense. I spent many an hour crying in his office in frustration as he kept explaining the legal ramifications of what I wanted to accomplish. He worked out the contract that I would need for the physician and myself. We discussed the fine line between the nursing practice and practicing medicine without a license. He shared court cases where other nurse practitioners had been sued. Every time I turned around there seemed to be another overwhelming challenge. Here I was trying to work and develop an idea with no clear direction. There was no mentor, only sixth sense of what I believed in. I was going to gamble, but what if I lost? I have never experienced a panic attack, but I can certainly empathize with women who have. My anxiety during those days was high. Somehow I survived all the attorney's dire predictions with a firm resolve to continue to pursue my dream.

Second, I had no concept of how to set up an office. In nursing school there were no business courses, and when I obtained my master's degree I did not take the ones that were available at UCLA; I opted for the teaching minor. So once again I was facing a great unknown. I didn't know about obtaining a business license or fire laws, etc. I began to look for an office so that I could have some sense of what my expenses would be. I hadn't saved to open my practice, so I honestly didn't know where I thought the money was going to come from.

I finally found a space on what we called "doctor's row." It was a disaster area. There were no sinks and the bathroom would have to be in the hallway. There were no walls, either, so those would have to be built. The amount of space I had was often referred to as my "midget office." Since I really didn't have much money I couldn't go into a fully designed space. I would have to improvise. My husband and friends began the enormous process of redesigning this space to make it resemble a medical office with all the necessities and none of the space. Walls were erected, sinks were put in, the space was rewired, the carpet was replaced, and somehow the dream was beginning to take form. The money to accomplish this came from my savings, a donation from my husband, and my friends working for free.

The biggest challenge remained. I still did not have a definite physician backup. Mark had agreed to back me up for a period of time, but I really needed a local gynecologist. I began with one of my physicians with whom I had worked. This presented a dual challenge. First, I realized that by discussing my dream, he might just fire me before I was ready to put my dream into a reality. Second, I would be taking some patients who had heretofore been seen in that office; therefore I would be affecting his revenue base to some degree. As one can imagine, my plan was met with disbelief and mixed emotions. We met in the office on a Sunday, and it was a feeling that one has when one party is asking for a divorce and the other partner has no idea. He promised to think about it. Just to complicate matters, we learned the next day that one of his employees had embezzled $10,000. To make things worse, the woman was someone I had recommended for the job. February of 1985 was certainly a month I will never forget. Eventually, after multiple meetings, negotiations, and with Mark's help, I received a commitment for one year.

After all of this I was exhausted. Remember, I still had no sense of how the women in the community would react. I needed them to be willing to believe in my dream. It never dawned on me what a challenge that would be. Perhaps that was best, because if I had known, would I have continued to pursue the dream? I suddenly realized that I wanted to make a living on high volume GYN. Women only have a pap smear once a year. I wanted to do patient education in an office setting. This was unheard of at that time. Most importantly, I was trying to do all this in a very conservative town that did not know what a nurse practitioner actually was. In my own ignorance, I didn't fathom that what I was trying to promote was a concept that was not being offered, by a type of healthcare professional that was unheard of, and in a town where the physicians would resent what I wanted to do.

The first step in the transition was sending out a note informing the women I had seen over the years that I was relocating. The second step was to begin being visible in the community. I began to speak in front of any organization which had any interest in women's health. Of course, these seminars were free, but it was a way to let women know who I was and what I wanted to do. The third step was having an open house. This legitimized my business. It demonstrated that I had nothing to hide. The open house was boycotted by all but three physicians in the community.

Once I had completed these tasks, I continued to network and maintain an active speaking schedule. I developed a lending library of books for women to borrow. I continued with the newsletter that I had started called *Women's Link to Health.* I was determined to make a difference.

Nothing prepared me for the disapproval which began to appear without warning. Sometimes it was an obvious comment, and sometimes it was more subtle. Many times prospective patients were told that I was not smart enough to get into medical school. Often times they were told that I was just a practicing nurse, so what could I know. And then there were the phone calls asking for Dr. Jones, so that I would get in trouble for practicing medicine without a license. The scariest incident was when I was reported to the state licensing board by one of the child psychiatrists in the community for using the term "counselor." Interestingly enough, the women in the community would come to their appointments despite the negative data.

Over time my practice continued to grow and evolve. I learned some specific marketing skills that worked and eliminated the ones that were not cost-effective. I began to surround myself with people who were creative and had the energy to dream. Every day I learned from the women I saw in my practice. I had taken a risk to believe in a dream, but that turned out to be just the first phase. There were so many steps in the process that there was no way of knowing. I lost $12,000 in the first year of my business. The overhead to open and maintain office equipment, insurance, and staff can be overwhelming. Because there was no mentor it was easy to make the wrong choices. There were moments when I just wanted to give up, and then I would receive a letter in the mail from someone whose life I had touched years ago, thanking me for caring.

As time passed the mistakes changed and the growth continued. My confidence in my dream grew, and slowly I realized that what had once been a dream was now a reality. I have now had my practice for six years here in the Ventura community. I continue to love and believe strongly in what I do, which is intrinsic for success.

People often ask me what I would do differently. The answer is complex. First, I would have paid more attention to my internal process. I have been a nurse for twenty years and I have always been a patient advocate. I was trying to improve the system. A part of me always wanted to do it "my way" but I didn't believe that was possible. I ignored my own sense of what could be if I was really willing to risk.

Second, I would have searched harder for a mentor. I thought that I needed to find someone who was doing exactly what I was doing. I was very active in women's rights, so I never looked at males as possible partial mentors. The whole concept of mentoring was not really well known then, but I never looked outside a select group.

Third, I would have talked to more people about my dream. I was afraid to share for a variety of reasons. If my dream never became a reality, fewer people would know. If I failed, I would have less explaining to do. I wondered: would people look at me with great skepticism and think I needed counseling? Sure, all those were possibilities—and at different times people did question my wisdom. Certainly there are still people who don't understand, and the big gest criticism has actually been from *nurses*. This was difficult to accept. It has taken time for people to understand that my dream is not a reflection on nursing. It is my interpretation of how I can use my skills as a nurse to help the most people.

What does the future hold for my dream? It is now at the age of menopause. We are looking at alternatives as the baby boomers go through the transition to the second half of their lives. This creates a great need for answers. Our teenagers are struggling with their sexuality and what this AIDS crisis means to them. The PMS controversy has never been resolved. There is much work that remains to be done. This is exciting! I have a vested interest in the menopause.

I have teenagers. I can continue to expand my dream.

I can only hope that as you have read this story, it provides you with the strength to believe in *you*. I want it to inspire in you the belief that almost anything is possible if you believe and if you work hard. Remember, you hold the key to your own dream.

Chapter 8

The Evolution of a Nurse Entrepreneur

by Gail Wick, RN,BSN,CNN

How does a nurse start and develop a business? How does one become a consultant? Neither question has a short, clear-cut answer, so let me share the evolution of my business and career with you as a stimulant for creative brainstorming.

In 1970, straight from nursing school, I jumped into what was emerging as an exciting specialty, nephrology nursing. I became a staff nurse in the renal ICU and transplant unit at Grady Hospital in Atlanta. After six months, I left the specialty for approximately three years, returning finally to become a staff nurse in the subspecialty of dialysis. Quickly, I subspecialized again as a teacher. I was first a home training instructor and later the education director for three large, nonprofit dialysis facilities in Atlanta. My specialty niches of nephrology nursing and teaching were created.

When I chose a specialty in nursing which I truly loved, found exciting, and which met the needs of a large healthcare consumer population, I began the development of what I now call the strategic plan for my career. Nephrology nursing with a focus on teaching became my first career path. All else would come from this focus. As part of the plan, I became very knowledgeable about my specialty and consistently worked to develop my teaching and lecturing skills. I read books, attended hundreds of seminars and meetings, and practiced what I learned on a regular basis.

I began to network at every opportunity. Through my attendance at meetings and networking opportunities, I chose role models to learn from, and developed a mentor relationship with a highly respected nephrology nurse, author, and teacher. Later, as I developed a serious interest in the business issues of healthcare, I found nurse/business person role models as well as non-nursing role models in the business world.

I joined professional organizations and actively worked on committees. Eventually I became an officer in many of them, thus increasing my visibility. Although I have a lot of volunteer time and effort, I gained as much or more than I gave. Through my involvement, I met my colleagues and the business people in my specialty, gained credibility as a specialist and, importantly, kept a pulse on the state-of-the-art and the needs of the specialty community.

I began speaking at meetings, first presenting abstracts, later as an invited speaker and seminar leader. For a long time I wasn't paid, but as time passed, my skills and uniqueness as a speaker enabled me to ask for compensation. This was in actuality the beginning of my consulting/education business, which I began officially in 1983. My business and marketing plans still call for speaking engagements because they provide income, exposure, and free marketing opportunities.

In the early 1980s I began to realize that I had a serious interest in not just the healthcare business, but business in general. This insight came from a number of sources. I began to work as a part-time consultant for a catheter company, and realized that I had a knack not just for teaching about the products, but also for selling the product. I didn't officially pursue sales as a career, but did begin to learn as much as possible about selling. I began to attend sales and business related seminars to develop the knowledge base I lacked. I observed sales and business people in as many settings as possible. I also focused on customer service and satisfaction, fee structuring and basic marketing principles. This knowledge base later helped me sell my company's services for a reasonable profit and keep my customers satisfied.

While I was testing the water of the corporate healthcare setting, I put another of my talents—designing—to work, and bought a small wholesale home decorative accessory business. I didn't make a lot of money, and I worked far too hard, but I gained valuable experience in marketing, sales, budgeting, management, and business partner relationships. Because I only focus on the positive aspects of the experience when I discuss that business, it has helped me gain credibility as a business person with my corporate clients today.

Today, my company is officially identified as Gail Wick & Associates, offering healthcare consulting, placement, and education services. Although many of my presentations and seminars have universal appeal, the consulting and placement services are specific to nephrology. We service both manufacturers and healthcare providers. Seminars and meeting management round out the education services.

The name of my company serves three main purposes—use of name recognition from years of visibility within my target market, identification of the company's primary focus, and flexibility to expand services and focus as opportunities arise. I believe that an entrepreneur must always be alert to exciting opportunities and needs which identify themselves in amazing ways. For the present, though, by concentrating on an area in which I am knowledgeable, known, and have an extensive network, I have been able to find a profitable niche quickly.

As I look to the future, I recognize a need to increase and refine my knowledge of the business of healthcare. Improved negotiation skills, more sophisticated marketing techniques, and development of a long-range business plan are immediate needs. Networking activities and involvement in organizations will become increasingly important. And perhaps most importantly, my commitment to nurse-owned organizations will continue to fuel my drive and commitment to nurse entrepreneurship!

From reading the above, it sounds like the development of my career path was very well thought out, smooth and calculated, doesn't it? Hardly! What you have read above is sixteen years of hindsight talking. The actual development of my career and current business was actually part luck, part accident, and part design.

Probably the best things that I have had going for me over the years are my true belief in what I'm doing, my love and respect for nursing and nurses, the insight to identify what I wanted from my career early, the ability to "fake it while I'm making it," and the guts to go for what I want.

Gail Wick & Associates
5420 New Wellington Close
Atlanta, GA 30327
(404) 252-9341

Chapter 9

Diversification and Determination: A Magic Formula

(This profile appeared in the November 1990 issue of the *Nurse-Entrepreneur's Exchange*.)

Editors Note: A few months after opening its doors for business in 1985, Lannie Liggett, RN, BSN, joined Analytical Medical Enterprises, Inc. (AME) of Baton Rouge, Louisiana as executive vice president.

AME started as a supplemental staffing agency run out of the home of president William F. Borne, RN. Today, AME has twenty-four offices in twelve states, and with 1990 revenues expected to approach $20 million, AME was the seventy-fifth fastest growing U.S. company last year according to **INC. Magazine.**

AME has also launched four other healthcare businesses in areas including contract anesthesia, physician office management, home health, and a traveling nurse company. It also owns a food catering service with its own seafood processing factory, along with a frozen food product line.

NEE: Tell us abut AME's corporate structure.
Lannie: "The people that run this business; the management, marketing, and clerical people are all employees. All of our nurses are

independent contractors because I think that nurses deserve the right to be independent. Not that every nurse should be independent—but they should have that option."

NEE: Have you had any encounters with the IRS?
Lannie: "Yes, often. They regularly show up and do compliance checks. They check the contracts, 1099s and other forms. We did request a private letter ruling status, but as of late 1989 the IRS quit issuing PLR's in nursing because they say it's a national issue. And at some point they will issue a national ruling."

NEE: AME has expanded into many areas. Describe these for us.
Lannie: "In 1987 we expanded the staffing business to include contract respiratory therapists.

That year we also opened General Anesthesia Services (GAS). This is the contract-anesthesia company which includes both MD's and CRNA's. Our CRNA's are paid a percentage of the billing, and the MD makes a percentage of whatever the CRNA does. The reason it's set up that way is because in our area hospital policy often requires that an MD be in the facility whenever a CRNA is giving anesthesia. So there's a billing split, but the CRNA makes much more than the MD, which is kind of a reverse. In our area, CRNA's are normally employees earning a set salary regardless of how much anesthesia they give. Now, for the first time in this area, because they are contracted, the CRNA makes a percentage of each case.

About the same time, we participated in the opening of Physician's Office Management, Inc., which provides accounting, bookkeeping, and personnel services to MD's in private practice.

I say *participated* because all of these other companies have other ownership besides AME. Although their businesses are housed in our corporate office, they all have separate management. These people all own stock in the company because we've always felt that the individuals who handle the business and make it grow need to have some ownership. So our people get a return in their salary as well as equity in the ownership."

NEE: Then you started Cajun A-La-Carte. How did that happen?
Lannie: "When AACN's National Teaching Institute convention came to New Orleans in 1987, we wanted to provide a hospitality event for the 4,000 participants. When we found out that catering costs would be $100,000 we decided to do it ourselves.

In order to do that, we had to buy a lot of catering equipment that we were unable to rent. With all of this equipment, we decided to start a business that catered authentic Cajun food to large companies— and it's been very successful.

Once we started catering, we go so many requests for the products themselves that we opened a USDA-certified kitchen and now produce a six-product frozen food line. It's called A-La-Carte Foods, and is sold in retail grocery stores in the U.S. and soon to be in Europe.

The kitchen we opened was located next to a seafood processing plant which was looking for expansion investment capital. So in early 1988, A-La-Carte Foods bought 40 percent of the plant so that we would have a close source of fresh seafood and get 40 percent of the equity in that company back on our balance sheets.

The catering business actually complements our nursing business in that we do a *Cajun Night* hospitality event at many State Nurse Association conventions every year. These are promotional events, and let me tell you, it works a lot better than classified ads!

In late 1988 we started Amedisys, our home health company, which presently services the state of Louisiana. In the future we plan to have an Amedisys office in every AME office.

Amerinurse, our traveling nurse division, opened in March of 1990 and is based in New Orleans. We're working on expanding Amerinurse to Europe, so it will eventually be international in scope."

NEE: All of this, and now you are a new mother as well!
Lannie: "Yes, I turned thirty-four, knew the biological clock was running, and I wanted to have a life with many facets—not just one. My whole adult life has been consumed with my career, and I felt that there were other areas of life that needed to be enjoyed, and having a child was one of those."

NEE: Any tips for nurses wanting to start a business?
Lannie: "Have more money than you need. You'll need two to three times as much as you think. Also, consider allowing other people to be an owner in your business. That keeps your early costs down because you get 'employees' for relatively little money. By giving them stock, it provides the incentive to put in the time and energy needed to make the company grow.

Also, it's hard to have other things in your life when you're starting out. If you're married, have kids—if you have a full bucket already—it makes it pretty tough unless you have a very understanding partner.

It takes sixteen to twenty hours a day to start a business, depending on what your level of success is. You have to make a decision on what it is that you're looking for. That will dictate how much time you need to spend. From the day I entered nursing school at seventeen, I knew I wanted to have a nursing role in business. I wasn't looking for $30,000 a year and a one-person operation. I was looking for the big time, so it was okay for me to devote my life to it and that's what I did."

Chapter 10

Maybe I Can...

by Cora LeClair, RN, CCRN

After my paycheck was cashed, taxes and bills paid, and with about $40 left, I thought: "Wow, maybe I can take a weekend trip (as long as I don't use too much gas, or stay in a motel, or eat in a restaurant...)."

Believe it or not, this was a common occurrence in my life about six years ago. I was lucky to bring home $800 every two weeks (working full-time as a staff nurse at a local hospital). With that money I paid my rent, living expenses, automobile payment, and insurance for my Mazda RX7. The car alone took over $500 each month! To be frank, I simply needed more money to live in Marin county, a beautiful place on the temperate California coast. I remember thinking to myself, how on earth do people afford to live here? Surely there must be nurses out there making less money than I who are apparently making it just fine. Or are they as poor as I am, and just not talking about it? As I cautiously approached my nursing friends, I discovered that the latter was indeed the case.

So I thought, why shouldn't I contract my own services rather than going through an agency or registry to do it for me? It can't be that difficult. There are so many talented individuals in the nursing business, why hasn't anybody thought of this yet? I saw a good many unhappy nurses out there who would be happy to contract themselves without using middlemen to control their careers for them. The best thing I could do for nursing at the time was to create a better way of offering nursing services—my own as well as others.

It seems like such a long time ago now; I had just finished a winter registry contract in Palm Springs, and I had been working all the hours I could stand, plus a little more. My car had expired, and my husband spent a weekend driving the eleven-hour trip to get me home. I felt physically and mentally exhausted. I just couldn't bear the thought of going out of town again to work. The area near my home offered none of the twelve-hour shifts I preferred. I arrived home anxious, moody, and feeling terribly unsettled.

I needed to have more control over my work life. I sat down at my desk and thought carefully about what I could change about my work. Perhaps I could still be happy being a critical care nurse! An idea took shape, and that day, with only $100 in my bank account, I began an endeavor that now brings me a salary of more than $100,000 annually.

This idea, you understand, was to see if I could work by professional contract at a hospital in much the same way as maintenance work, construction, and doctor's services are done. I would save management the cost of administration, accounting and benefits, just as the registries do; the hospital in turn, would pay me substantially more than a regular staff nurse and still save money. I contacted hospitals in my area to see if they needed help in their ICU's. I queried registries and traveling nurse agencies and found out where hospitals were short of staff. I made a few more calls and soon found a little town in Northern California desperately needing a critical care nurse for January.

So I packed my bags with two weeks worth of professional and play clothes and devised my first contract for services. Then I drove the three hours required to get there and presented myself and my contract to the Director of Nurses. I was asked to start right away, and could I please work that night?

It was that simple. I got an apartment, plunged into my work, kept all my receipts and invoices for tax records, and quickly found several other nurses who were keenly interested in starting their own businesses just the way I did. In no time, I was teaching others on a consultant basis and collecting a very fair fee for my services. I perfected my contracts with the help of a business lawyer, obtained a good bookkeeper and an accountant who specialized in small businesses. I even created a publication about contracting nursing services so that others could follow the same simple steps I had taken to begin their ventures. Nurses were soon hearing about my business from word-of-mouth, advertisements, and by my self created brochures.

It wasn't long after I started circulating brochures that I was asked to speak at the 1990 National Nurses in Business Association conference. I had always enjoyed public speaking but figured I had better brush up on a few techniques. Besides, how could I mess up talking about something I really enjoyed and truly believed in? I agreed to speak, knowing it would also be a great opportunity to meet other nurses who were trying new ideas and starting out in business. In finding out about the NNBA, I had finally discovered an entire group of nurses who were also entrepreneurs, just like me. Witnessing the creativity and self-power of the people attending this conference, I became certain that the concept of directing one's own career as a business held the brightest future for nursing professionals.

My company, now nearly six years in existence, is officially called LeClair Enterprises, and is located in a small city in central Marin county. I continue to perform nursing services myself through private hospitals by contract and consult with nurse-clients to design contracts and draft resumes. In the last two years, I have become a professional contract negotiator for individuals and nursing registries. This is a new, wide-open field which still holds untapped areas of resources and income for anyone interested.

61

Tips for success? Start your business in your home and have a room designated as your office. Carry regular office hours, just as if you had to report to an employer. You will find it tempting at first to try to mix in domestic work; a little vacuuming and dusting or a little laundry. Don't! Remember, you will be doing all the things your administrator used to do for you; i.e. arranging your benefits, withholding your taxes, and keeping records. It may seem like an easy job, but record keeping may be too taxing and time consuming to accomplish yourself. My opinion is this: let the experts do what they are educated to do.

You need the time spent in your office to accomplish the tasks at hand. Don't let your business life become chaotic and disorganized. Otherwise, you will find stepping into your home office to be a drudgery, and you will have difficulty getting things done. Keep the experience a positive one. This realization came to me in a desperate moment of reckoning, after which I began to work in my office from noon to five, Monday through Friday. Be realistic, and set hours that fit your schedule with some room for flexibility.

A computer, a printer, a good file cabinet, and a desk are essential furnishings in the office of any professional, along with a business line to keep your business calls separate, and an answering machine. The computer need not be very fancy or super modern. The older PC-compatible type can be found used for very little money. If you are a true friend to yourself, buy one with a hard disk drive of any size. Obtain a dot matrix printer and word processing software. Now you are off and running! Later you will find a data base program very helpful, but don't worry about that at first. You can buy a wonderful array of "how to" books at any bookstore to teach yourself how to use a computer. Or, perhaps it would be more worth your effort to take some computer classes at a local college. These are usually very economical.

If you are planning to start a registry, you should have least $150,000 in reserve, as hospitals usually pay these agencies on a 90-day turnaround basis. If you will have partners, pick them carefully, and consult an attorney before committing yourself to any partnership. Design your contracts to have a penalty for late payment. A two percent discount for on-time payment is a standard policy in business.

You will need a business or contract lawyer to look over your potential contracts for you. There is nothing worse than having a contract signed and, later, realizing that you left something very important out. You will do a lot of praying until that contract is up, just hoping nothing goes wrong. Hire a tax accountant and bookkeeper. Pick people who are sympathetic to your business ideas. There are naysayers out there who, with great hubris, will say you can't do this and you're asking for serious trouble. Skip over these people! Negative energy never got you to this point in your business. I also used an organizational consultant who showed me ways to file documents efficiently, how to precisely organize accounting work, and even helped me on my brochure. These professionals may seem expensive, but they are worth it. No successful business can last long without their services.

Last, but certainly not least, try not to let the day-to-day financial strains get to you. Your own business is better evaluated on a yearly basis, rather than looking at the brief high and low cycles alone. It helps to have a good friend or business associate be your shoulder to cry on during stressful times. You will probably remember your first year in business for yourself as one in which you were terribly poor, but one you would live all over again to reap the rewards that lie ahead!

Chapter 11

Pure, Unadulterated Frustration

by Imalee Crow, RN

Associate Medical Professionals (AMP), an agency specializing in solving hospital staffing problems, was born out of pure, unadulterated *frustration.*

For ten years I had worked as a hospital nurse administrator/manager, and then as an administrator for three different agencies. I knew what hospitals and nursing supervisors were asking for. Although each agency I had worked for had every chance for success, these companies had instead chosen to push a product instead of listening to the client. In each company, I was asked to be responsible for everything, but I had only the authority related to the clinical side of nursing, with no control over the business side.

The result? No one was winning! The hospital clients, the agency, and I—no one was meeting the goals. And the most frustrating thing was that it didn't have to be that way—I *knew* how to solve those problems.

Today, after a lot of planning and hard work, my own company is meeting needs for hospitals and nurses, and making a profit for our agency. I've never been happier or more fulfilled. Not only is AMP operating on a win-win-win philosophy, we are seeing that our company is changing the image of agency nursing. And, we are a part of a new attitude of pride that is rebuilding Oklahoma.

With encouragement from my husband, I resigned from the agency. He wisely pointed out what I couldn't see alone—that I already had a foot in every hospital door in town.

At the time I decided to go into business, Oklahoma was in severe economics times; the bottom had just dropped out of the oil market, Penn Square Bank had folded, and the outlook for new businesses was bleak. But my husband, Chuck, assured me that my broad understanding of hospitals and my organizational abilities, combined with the need for nurses throughout the city, was enough to build a successful company. "Besides," he said, "you have personal credibility within every nursing department in town, and with my salary we'll make it fine."

Once we decided to move forward, the first thing we did was develop a written business plan complete with a budget, time line, analysis of the competition, and projections for the first year. The budget provided a modest salary for me from the beginning, to free me from panic. I knew myself well enough to know that without some personal compensation early on, I could easily panic and give up before the company had time to develop.

We also planned from the beginning to advertise every week, without fail, in order to develop and keep a pool of qualified nurses. Since the first week, we have been consistently in the Sunday classifieds—advertising our distinction, our benefits, and our pay.

A computer, too, was included in the budget. Since there was no other office staff for the first three months (I was it!), we knew that a computer would be vital for correspondence, placement, payroll, and billing. In addition, we used my experience to develop a computer program for maintaining a roster of qualified RN's and LPN's. The experience of each person on our staff is stored in our computerized retrieval system, so we can quickly locate particular nurses with special experience to match the client's needs.

Next, we received a line of credit through a small CD and got a business loan by placing a second mortgage against our home. By August of 1987, we had every form created, every pencil in place, and held an open house to let the world know we were in business.

We opened with three hospital contracts. But we knew from the beginning that regular communication with these clients was vital to our success. I told clients that although AMP nurses would serve them as agreed, clients would not be seeing me for three months. I showed them our game plan and why it would take me full-time to market our services to the other hospitals in order to be a successful agency. I also shared with them the benefits of working with me and how we could all *win* by working together.

This planning and commitment to marketing, combined with our own good service, has really paid off. Since then, the company has grown to three full-time office employees, fifteen client hospitals throughout the state, and $2 million in annual gross billings. We are serving all types of clients, all shifts in all areas, including: Psychiatric, ICU, ER, OR, CCU, Labor and Delivery, Nursery, Rehab, Recovery Room and Med/Surg. Our clients range in size from 600-bed metropolitan hospitals to under 100-bed rural hospitals, as well as specialty clinics.

However, the last three years have not all been smooth and sweet. I'll never forget the day they walked in and served me with those legal papers—an icy-cold fear gripped my heart, and I thought about dying right there on the spot. You see, within three weeks after we opened our doors, we received notice that we were being sued for a huge amount of money by my former employer for what the legal beagles called a "violation of non-compete clause." The stress and legal expense that followed were, to say the least, unpleasant. And all of this was when I needed to focus on building a business.

As it turned out, a client-hospital friend was able to help close out the deposition against us, and the charge was dropped. At every place of employment, I had been careful not to take files, lists, or forms, except for those I had personally developed. Fortunately, in Oklahoma the non-compete is very hard to enforce and seldom holds up in court. But until it was all over, I found difficulty sleeping, eating, or working.

Then, only a few months later, my husband's "secure" job was eliminated, and more stress was added to our lives. Dealing with the emotional and financial strain on top of trying to build a fledgling company was very tough—to say the least. But again, the planning and hard work paid off. By March of that year, Chuck was added to the payroll here at the company. He took the responsibility for the computer processing, advertising, and miscellaneous tasks that were becoming overwhelming for me.

We offer both contract staffing (PAC's or Planned Assignment Contracts) and per diem staffing. Our company's day-to-day performance is based on a belief in excellence, problem solving, accountability, and giving. We have a written statement of this philosophy which hangs on the wall for all to see.

A key element to our success, I believe, has been our "paper trail" for clients. We put everything in writing. We have guaranteed service, and we put our name on the line in a certificate to each client. We developed and copyrighted the JCAHO Nurse Profile, which gives clients a complete record of each nurse's experience, credentials, and records. Every procedure, standard, and job description is in writing. This gives great confidence to our clients—particularly when they face accreditation teams.

We also utilize the AMP FAX to give instant response to client needs (and save us time traveling). Our company offers 24-hour service and Two-Hour Check-In (a nurse verification) before shifts begin. Even our AMP Performance Correction Reports are in writing to follow up on complaints. We have been able to solve every problem by discussing it, dealing with it, and documenting it clearly. In short, we have developed each program to meet client concerns.

One area of vital concern to clients is the billing process. Our system of AMP Value Billing utilizes the computer to clearly give supervisors all the information needed for rapid reconciliation. It offers individual entries, location-cost breakdown, attached copies of original numbered tickets for reference, and a summary of hourly charges. In our list of references, we are proud to have financial coordinators as well as nurse supervisors. Our clients tell us AMP billing is reconciled in one-third the time compared to other agency's bills.

Another critical factor to growth has been our ability to keep quality nurses. It was not just the weekly advertising which has cultivated this pool. We developed top pay, travel expenses, and written criteria-based job descriptions. AMP has daily pay, excellent benefits, the AMP Nurse Forum (a semi-annual professional exchange), TOP 100 (a professional nurse and customer development program), AMP Nurse Apartment (free accommodations for out-of-town nurses working two or more shifts), Quality Check (an on-site quality assessment program), monthly birthday recognition, fun contests, and TOP 1,000 (recognition for those working 1,000 hours or more). All these have been developed because the nurses asked and we listened.

All our employees have our respect. We tell them how important they are, we encourage them to improve, and we expect the best performance. But, I, believe, the primary reason our employees stay in line is that we listen to them. They believe we need them to help make decisions for the company, and we do! Our employees are our partners.

In 1989, we added a marketing consultant to our staff in order to get more visibility out of the programs we had already developed. Our client newsletters have helped tell our story. We mail these to current and prospective clients throughout the state, as well as to our own nursing staff. One of the nicest benefits have been the client testimonials. It is encouraging to hear from clients who tell the world why they use AMP. Some clients have even *asked* to be interviewed for the newsletter. What an opportunity!

The marketing consultants have given us a regular "outside/inside" view of ourselves providing clarification and insight. The regular feedback from a professional has been very helpful. Using materials we already had, we now have phonehold messages, paycheck inserts, employee newsletters, *The Nurse Journal*, and visuals for TOP 100 and Quality Check. In addition, marketing expertise helped us with newspaper advertising, corporate sales, and recruitment materials.

Recently I was asked if having your own business is worth the risk. My answer is definitely yes! The fulfillment of creating a business, of meeting needs for hospitals and nurses, is incredibly satisfying. And our income has never been better.

But the whole process has taught me. I've learned that I couldn't do it alone. I needed my husband to share the risk with me. Although I manage the business, his expertise is a real asset, and we couldn't make it without that. Chuck has also been my emotional "safety valve." I can count on him to help keep me balanced; he knows just when I need to get away and refocus. I have also learned that nurses *can* be successful businesspeople. However, the business side must be learned; just caring isn't enough to run a business.

Another important lesson has been the value of planning. It was the initial planning which got us the loan and carried us through those first months. Without a plan, I would have caved in with the sheer weight of the problems we encountered. The plan let our clients see we were going somewhere, let others help us, and let us see the vision of success.

Ongoing planning has been a part of our company. It has become part of our philosophy, allowing us to stay ahead of JCAHO mandates, and allowing us to offer support to client hospitals that is just not a step, but miles ahead.

Associate Medical Professionals
4801 N. Classen Blvd., Suite 208
Oklahoma City, OK 73118
(405) 842-0003

Chapter 12

How to Doughnut-Proof a Nurse

by Joan Downey, RN, and Margaret Freidin, RN

Reading lips obscured by tape and surrounding tubefilled mouths was not our strong suit, nor that of anyone else we met; that's why we started the Silent Speaker.

This inability seemed widespread, not something we had a monopoly on. However, nothing was being done to help those who really needed it—the patients. When one of our patients almost lost his eyesight because none of us involved in his care could understand him, we decided to develop a tool for the patients' use. The original Silent Speaker actually took its first breaths the night I realized that this young man wanted to say "blurry," but it would be a couple of years before it could stand on its own.

As originally conceived, the Silent Speaker consists of the anatomical forms, anterior and posterior, and words allowing communication of urgent or essential needs. It was printed directly onto clipboards so that they could carry a conversation as well as papers and earn their keep instead of just hanging around.

The concept eventually expanded to include not only clipboards but laminated cards of clipboard size, pocket-sized cards, posters, and tear-off sheet tablets. These tablets were designed to be included in every desk drawer and admission pack so that persons with actual or threatened communication problems can have their say. In addition to products in English, there were bi-lingual versions and some alowing for any second language to be added. But this was all down the road.

Margaret and I had worked together in the ICU for a few years on nights, then evenings and days. Our friendship was built on innate grit, integrity, and humor which spilled into our nursing care, and were essential ingredients in establishing the business and seeing it through.

The original Silent Speaker was copyrighted by me, and while waiting for this Oz-like seal to arrive from the government, I realized that I didn't have the foggiest idea how to do what I was doing; that is, put essential words and phrases on a clipboard. The one I made utilized rub-on letters that I purchased at the stationery store. The attorney almost rubbed them off as he examined the clipboard. Faced with knowing that I didn't know what to do or how to do it, it seemed logical to approach Margaret to join me in these uncharted waters. The grit kicked in immediately, and she said something that I've repeated hundreds of times since: "In for a penny, in for a pound."

One of the first things we noticed was the number of words that formally meant nothing and now meant business, such as: business license, fictitious name, tax number, trademark, minimum quantity, purchase order, 30-day net. We had walked into another world. There is no doubt in either of our minds that without the discipline, determination, and ingenuity required as nurses we'd have never stuck it out.

On the advice of the attorney, we created several designs and copyrighted those. We attempted to find white clipboards—outside of two at yard sales, we never did. After exhausting more than 100 companies and printers, all of whom said they couldn't print on clipboards because the ink came off, Margaret located one who said he could do it.The boards were thick, brown, and had to be hand cut. The clips were massive, capable of hanging up a week's laundry, and pop-riveted in place by hand. One clipboard cost $85.00, which presented a bit of a marketing problem, but I doubt anything short of our kids' births caused us a more delight.

In the light of day it looked awful, the artwork shakily hand-drawn and words typed on an ancient typewriter, but it had a beauty that our labor and love had endowed to it. The printer then informed us that he only had enough material to make 500 clipboards and that he only had ten clips. So we began the great clipboard-clip hunt again.

Jim and Paul, our spouses, went on wild goose chases all over Southern California in search of this elusive material. In desperation, we decided to try shower walls. It had some merit using a different printing technique, so we cut up the "minimum purchase" into a couple of hundred boards. We learned what we could about pop-riveting. Meanwhile, our printer left town.

Remember *grit*, as this was just the beginning.

We ordered business cards. The printer wanted our artwork, so, while leaning on the counter, I drew him our logo, the human forms without a mouth, depicted on a clipboard under a clip. When we picked up our 1,000 business cards (remember bulk) we were saddened because of the cost, but amused to see that our logo-man looked like he was hanging from a coat hanger instead of standing under a clip. Coupled with our other artwork, this fact led us to a graphic artist. We'd never known what they did, but if it's something you read or look at, odds are a graphic artist has had a hand in it. (We subsequently trademarked our logo-man and our company name, Silent Speaker.)

Saved by the bell! Or so it seemed, when a large company claimed to want to help small, women/minority-owned businesses and accepted our request for assistance. They almost helped us right out of business. They manufactured clipboards for us and then went on to make laminated cards which we decided to do for infectious disease cases, and to expand availability and make good on our commitment to have this available to all who needed it.

Excited with our good fortune, we sold products to hospitals and booked our first major exhibit at a nursing conference in Las Vegas in February of 1988. On December 29th, I received a call from this company's representative informing me that we needed to purchase in bulk. Our costs had been escalated from test market quantities of twenty-five to a hundred pieces, to numbers that raised our minimum order into the $20,000 price range.

We were shattered! A lawsuit, though logical, was out of the question because although operating alone, a member of one of our families was employed by this company. Much was at stake besides the business.

Daunted but determined, and relying more on prayer than the phone book, we headed out once again to find help—and found it almost under our noses. A gentleman in town had a business that specialized in the unusual, and he said he'd help find a manufacturer. Meanwhile, we leaned on the other company to supply what we needed to see us through the commitments we had made, and they did.

We went to Las Vegas, loading the van with tables, chairs, silk flowers and vases, and dozens of Silent Speakers, with the idea of setting up a first-class booth. By the way, booths are very expensive. What we didn't do is read the fine print. One can take into the exhibit hall only that which one person can carry and set up in under fifteen minutes, much like a business marathon. We arrived with enough to set up house. With the blessings of one of the exhibit directors who sensed our newness and lack of revenue, Margaret, my husband, Jim, and I hauled our inventory into the convention hall.

Getting out, or torn down as they say, was even more exciting. When they announce that an exhibit is over, they aren't kidding. The carpets are rolled up almost before the announcement is over. We were almost impaled on forklifts and crushed by trucks as, sweat-soaked, we carried our borrowed furniture out into the snow and rain and loaded the van, dressed in suits and high heels, except Jim, who had sense enough to stick with low shoes.

The exhibit was exhilarating; nurses knew what the product was for, and it sold itself. The sense of accomplishment was intoxicating. But we were to learn another hard lesson, namely that nurses who needed this for their patients were not necessarily the ones who decided how to spend the budget dollars. That same budget that would pay nurses to play charades with the patient, that would allow the outcome of the illness to be worse than it would have been, and to heaven only knows what degree—*death* being a possibility—that same budget would not necessarily include funds for a Silent Speaker.

Business is reality, Goliath lives, and one must learn to use a slingshot. Miraculously, our new contact found a company that made nothing but printed clipboards, and we ended up with a much better product. Finding a laminator was almost as hard, as most couldn't provide the thickness we wanted so that the product would be durable.

In the last two years, we have exhibited our products nationally and met thousands of people, mostly nurses. The Silent Speaker has been well received and appreciated for its simplicity, light weight, and low cost. We have enjoyed a renewed sense of pride in ourselves for utilizing the problem-solving skills we had internalized in nursing and also developed a deep kinship with fellow nurses who want to take themselves, and their profession, forward.

Probably the most sobering statement about nurses was made to us while exhibiting at a fairly large event. The man next to us was a medical products distributor. We complimented him on one of his products; disposable, paper baby scrub gowns. He thanked us and then called us closer to share a secret. He got the idea for this, his best seller, from nurses. He said all the good ideas came from nurses and that if we wanted to know anything we should ask a nurse. "They have the best ideas; they'll tell you everything about it and give it away. They're happy if you bring them a dozen doughnuts." We smiled and said, "Really."

On the way home we dissected his words. They were *true*. How many times had we seen doctors throw fits, then assuage the damage with an annual donation of doughnuts. Or, how many times had we improvised a piece of equipment only to see it later marketed.

Margaret and I had earned a reputation at work as being "doughnut proof" before we ever started this venture, and after the man's comments, harsh as they were, we realized that it was this sense of self-worth that had taken us this far. We strongly encourage nurses we meet to develop their own ideas and *never* give them away. If you don't believe in yourself, no one else will either.

Probably the hardest lessons we've learned continue to be played out while we write this story. There is the possibility of a large company taking our idea and then having to follow up on their action. And there is the constant swimming against the tide dealing with companies because we aren't ordering thousands of items with each order. Many businesses just aren't interested in doing business with a small company. Bulldog-like, one has to bite and hang on and demand that deadlines be met, products supplied, bills paid. The business people that have helped us, and for the most part that means doing what they are paid to do and doing it well, have our respect and our business.

We have had to continue working in nursing, because we took on another job with the business and were never relieved of the one we already had as major contributors to our own families' support. Until this year, I did most of the office work and shipping. Now, my daughter handles the office, and Jim does the shipping. This help has been an enormous relief.

In undertaking this venture, we had no idea that the bullet we would be biting was a cannon shell. This is not a world for the faint-hearted or for those who have to know the outcome before they begin. There is, however, a sense of real accomplishment knowing that we have done what we set out to do and are fulfilling the unspoken promise to that patient who inspired us; that we would do all in our power to ensure that every patient had the opportunity to express his needs if he was in any way able to do so.

If you've always wanted to know what adrenaline tastes like, looks like, and feels like, go into business.

UPDATE 1997

It hardly seems possible that six years have passed since I wrote the article for *"How I Became a Nurse Entrepreneur,"* yet much has happened in that time.

The spirit that enabled Margaret and me to develop the Silent Speaker is the same spirit that sends nurses into the unknown daily, where life blood pours out and hearts beat chaotically on death's door and complaints must be sifted for their relevance...or else. It is this spirit that has sustained us during adverse times.

In the original article, when I mentioned a large company taking our idea, it was a reality, not a what if. We had met one of their representatives at an exhibit and he was so enthusiastic about including the

Silent Speaker with each of their speciality beds. Unfortunately, he presented the idea to his company as his own, and they "loved it!" When we re-met him, he gushed over their success. They had printed our information and figures using different colors with the text rearranged, and were giving them away with the same freedom one passes out business cards. We were forced to hire attorneys to try to stop them. In reply, the company did exactly what our copyright attorney predicted: they claimed a nurse "in Texas" gave them the idea. We wondered if they gave her a dozen donuts or perhaps, hushpuppies?

Wallowing in self-pity or anger is something neither Margaret or I tolerate and we continued to present the Silent Speaker across the country. We consistently received enthusiastic comments from fellow nurses, although we would occasionally meet some who spoke of the one "just like" ours that that company had given to them.

It was most encouraging to see the Silent Speaker accepted by the non-professional community as evidenced by the positive responses from families we met at meetings and exhibits centered on ALS or Muscular Dystrophy.

At a large nursing conference in the East, we introduced our product line to Harry Tiggard, Jr., President of Trademark Medical. He was impressed and agreed to take some samples and exhibit them at other conferences. He found as we had, that nurses knew what they were and wanted them.

Somewhere along the line, I started to not feel up to par and learned that hepatitis I had contracted from an earlier needlestick had become chronic, leaving my enzymes elevated and my energy low. Subsequently, I was forced to leave work in the ICU. Major life changes, the kind I had often talked so reassuringly about to patients, had now come down to me.

Not having reached the point where we worked on the Silent Speaker, but also working in ICU as well, Margaret and I realized that we could no longer run our company to its fullest potential. We were pleased to have the opportunity to enter into an agreement with Mr. Triggard, at Trademark Medical, and his company has since been marketing the Silent Speaker. We have occasion to talk to the people at Trademark Medical on the phone and although we have only met a couple of them in person, all are friendly, cheerful and a pleasure to be associated with.

Margaret now works in open heart and enjoys being preceptor to nurses new to this area and to nursing students during their rotation. I work part time with persons who have cerebral palsy and oversee their health needs, develop care plans and write our newsletter. While we no longer envision taking something from infancy and rearing it through all the stages involved in growth on our own, we continue to be of like minds and from time to time submit ideas for consideration as new products. Running a business demands a ton of energy!

We belive that the Silent Speaker has yet to reach its potential. In a world that values communication, it is still the norm to find people guessing what someone on a ventilator is trying to say. It is still the norm to hear someone ask for an interpreter or state in great frustration that they can't understand "what you're trying to say" as they try to gather urgent information. In the February 1995 issue of *RN* magazine there was an article entitled "If Ventilator Patients Could Talk." It suggested using items for communication that have been proven not to work: children's erasable slates and scratch pads. I wrote a letter to the editor in which I expressed my sadness at the failure to grow in communication, and asked as Margaret and I have so many times, the following questions related to communication:

1. How can you meet your patients' needs if you don't know what they are?

2. How can you measure lost communication if you don't know what they are?

81

3. Could better communication have eased someone's pain, altered the course of an illness, saved a life?

I received no reply. It has been our experience that individual nurses appreciate the Silent Speaker for its ability to meet the needs of those unable to speak and of those unable to speak English. They purchase the Silent Speaker for their own use, and yet it would seem that hospitals would insist that all means possible be used to improve patient care, particularly in the area of communication, and would stock Silent Speakers. We look forward to this eventuality. We firmly believe that every hospital unit, emergency room, clinic, ambulance, school, airport, cruise ship would benefit by using the Silent Speaker clipboards, laminated card, wall charts, and pocket aides.

We developed the Silent Speaker to help people. We believe in it. It has demonstrated its worth and as our logo says, "it speaks for those who can't speak for themselves."

The Silent Speaker is available from:

Trademark Corporation
1053 Headquarters Park
Fenton, MO 63028-2033
(800) 325-3044

Chapter 13

Watching The Lights Go On

by Judith C. Miller, RN MS

I was up to my elbows in diapers and busy chasing toddlers, teaching Saturday nursing classes at a local university, and trying to decide what I wanted to do when I grew up when I was asked to tutor a student who had failed state boards.

What a job! I studied ten hours for every hour I tutored. But what fun! Working one-to-one is every educator's dream. Watching the "lights go on" in the learner turns on a teacher. I loved it. The student passed! Then came another request—and another. In those days I scheduled tutoring sessions late in the afternoon so I could get a high school baby-sitter.

After several successes, I decided there was a need for tutors and that I was good—very good—at meeting that need. I wrestled long and hard with the decision to advertise. Was it ethical? With sweaty palms I called the local newspaper and placed a three-lined ad. The phone started ringing, and the students started coming.

I continued to raise my children, teach part-time, and tutor for boards. This satisfied my needs to remain active professionally and be a full-time mother. I kept telling myself that I spent all that time, money, and energy earning a master's degree, and I certainly wanted to put it to use. Then tragedy struck—my husband was killed in an accident. I was left with three children, ages six and under. Fortunately, I was able to continue my part-time teaching, research and tutoring.

I was newly remarried when my youngest daughter started school. I increased my teaching, tutoring, and started teaching state board reviews and conducting test-taking workshops for a nurse who owned a review business. I still didn't know what I wanted to do when I grew up.

I knew that I did not want to be a permanent part of the university scene. I had taught at both two- and four-year nursing programs and did not like the "administrivia," the pettiness, and the infighting for tenure, but I loved to teach. As a part-time faculty member, I realized that I was used and abused. They would take everything I had to give—design a new course, revise this, etc., but I was getting nothing except the "personal rewards" of a job well done.

I decided to give myself a name, get another phone line, print some stationery and business cards and remodel the study for my home office. Nursing Tutorial and Consulting Services was born. I knew what the tutorial part was, but I had only a vague dream what the consulting part would become. I only knew I didn't want to limit myself.

As the student load began to fill all available hours, I realized that group classes would be a more efficient and more financially rewarding way to teach. By now I was an expert. So I rented a room in a church to teach small group classes two evenings a week. County ordinances did not allow more than five persons at a time to come to my home for business purposes. By this time I had graduated from a manual typewriter to a computer, a copier, and an answering machine in my office.

The decision to enter the business world in a big way was difficult. I had to move out of the house in order to grow. In the past, my husband and I had invested in residential rental real estate. It seemed natural to buy office space and rent out what I did not need. That way I would have room to grow when the time came. (My husband thought buying office space was strictly an investment, and my being there was incidental.) I set four criteria for my office investment:

1) public transportation must be available
2) easy access from major highways
3) space for a classroom as well as an office
4) zoning that would allow retail sales (I wanted to sell review books to my students).

I finally found the space. How scary it was to sign the papers! Could I rent out space to help pay the mortgage? Would my business grow? The office was mortgaged, and now my residence had a second mortgage. Suddenly, I realized this was for *real*.

My youngest daughter was proud of me and thought I must be a success because I had a drinking fountain in my office. My husband couldn't understand why I put "Rent Room" on both bathrooms and not "Men" and "Women".

The students came. My course offerings increased. I no longer had time for part-time teaching at the university. Hooray! I even needed help with the mounds of paper work. After a call to a high school guidance department, I soon had a delightful young student working after school typing, copying, etc.

I had to evict the first office tenant I had, a personnel agency, because he did not pay his rent. When I needed a part-time secretary, I called him and said, "Tony, get me a good secretary and I won't take you to court for the money you owe me." He sent over a wonderful young college student named Stephanie for me to interview. Three years and a bachelor's degree later she is still with me—now as my full-time administrative assistant and book store manager. I thought the loss of the tenant was difficult, but the trade-off was better. Stephanie is worth more to me than his rent ever could have been.

As my business grew, the demands on Stephanie increased. After particularly stressful times during which she exhibited great responsibility and initiative, I have given her raises. There were times when I wondered if I could afford to raise her pay, but I did, and she became very loyal. She started using the pronouns *we* and *us* when describing the business. I had a few uneasy moments when she graduated from college with a BA in Business Administration and started looking for full-time employment. She accepted my offer and has not disappointed me. She is growing with the business. In addition to her duties as administrative assistant and office manager, she manages the bookstore with very little guidance from me. Good support staff has been essential to the growth of my business.

My reputation grew. I became known as an expert on state boards, test writing, test taking, and helping international nurses pass the boards. The local colleges started sending me students who were having difficulty making it through the nursing program. I started doing educational consulting and writing. Doors began to open.

For a while, I continued to do reviews and workshops for the nurse-owned review business I had been working for. One day the owner said, "Judy, I don't want you to tell people that you tutor or do anything except work for me." Until that time, I had carefully structured my activities in a way that did not compete with her. When schools for which I had done workshops for her business started approaching me as an individual, I carefully referred them back to her. Needless to say, I no longer work for her and therefore no longer limit my scope. Severing this restrictive relationship freed me to realize my full potential. Any worries I had about losing that income vanished quickly as I expanded my activities. That year I made more money than ever before.

Another chance event launched a new business venture. I was asked to teach a certification review course. The sponsoring consortium wanted to videotape the review for consortium members throughout their state. Realizing that if they needed the review on videotape, so might other hospitals across the country. I offered to exchange my services for a master copy of the videotapes and rights to market the tape in the other forty-nine states. That was in 1989.

In 1990, I put out three new videotape review series (a total of twenty-eight tapes) and have more underway. The first tapes were in areas in which I could personally be the presenter. Now I am producing and marketing videotapes using other nurse experts. I offer the presenters a choice of cash payment for services or royalties. They all choose royalties, as well they should. It is better for them in the long run and, I think, better for me. They will promote the tapes if they have a direct financial interest.

What did I, a nurse, know about marketing and advertising? Not much. I was off to workshops and seminars for crash courses on entering the real world of business. Our county has wonderful adult education offerings. These were invaluable to me. The National Nurses in Business Association conferences the last two years have been sources of helpful information and inspiration.

I'll never forget the first time someone called me an *entrepreneur*. I was serving on a statewide nursing committee. The chairperson, a respected nurse educator, started enthusiastically introducing me to others as a successful nurse entrepreneur. Until that time, I felt that most of my nursing colleagues thought I was a little strange and not really a true nursing professional. I began to proudly claim the title of full-time nurse entrepreneur.

Turning adversity into opportunity and being willing to take risks have been the mainstays of developing my business. What a long way I have traveled —from sweaty palms placing a three-line ad in a local paper to masterminding national direct mail advertising campaigns and exhibiting at conventions; from an occasional student to speaking at national conferences and even overseas; from $10 an hour to a six-figure gross; from uni-focused teaching to a multipronged business; from a manual typewriter to an office with four computers, 1.5 full-time support staff, and seven part-time nurse consultants.

The ideas for growth keep coming. My problems now are deciding which endeavor to do first and what I can get others to do for me. I currently have four major foci: Tutoring and review classes; consulting and workshops primarily in the area of test construction and test taking; development and marketing of videotape reviews for certification exams and NCLEX; and a full-service nursing bookstore. I guess I'm still not sure I know what I want to do when I grow up, but I'm having fun trying to find out.

Has it been easy? No. I work more hours for me than I ever would for anyone else. Taking risks has become easier as I have had successes. I still swallow hard when I take a leap and start another new venture. Delegating is getting easier. When I first started out I had to do it all, because there was no one else. Now I am learning how to work through others. My personal guidelines are to always work professionally and with integrity in whatever I attempt. My husband and children do not always understand what I am doing, but they are supportive and understanding.

Has it been worth it? Yes, emphatically yes! Would I do it again? Yes, I love what I do, and I do what I love. What more could I ask for?

UPDATE 1997

Was it only six years ago I wrote "Watching the Lights Go On?" In some ways it seems like eons ago and in some ways it seems like yesterday.

The children are grown now and the cycles of life are turning. I am still doing business as Nursing Tutorial and Consulting Services. I still prepare nurses for NCLEX-RN and NCLEX-PN exams and tutor nursing students. I still produce and sell videos and have a small nursing bookstore. From time to time I have changed the product and service mix. I have added faculty workshops and am co-editor of a major NCLEX-RN book.

What have I learned in the past few years?

Life goes in circles. Six years ago I wrote about moving out of the house. I am now making plans to return my base of operations to my home. I am learning what works and what doesn't and how I want to spend my time. The children have grown and most are away from home. Commuting gets harder and harder and makes less and less sense. Cutting overhead costs by eliminating the office, doing administrative work from home and renting classroom space when needed, seem to make a lot of sense. I am now doing more "custom" reviews- "have overheads, will travel"- and workshops for faculty. These do not require expensive office space.

Learn from your mistakes or let go of non profitable ideas. Expanding the nursing bookstore beyond meeting the needs of the students who come to review classes is not cost-effective. The bookstore is expensive to run and requires either a huge volume or raising prices beyond recommended retail in order to be a money maker. I am not willing to do the latter and the former is not realistic. We now keep a limited stock of books on hand and special order other items.

Look before you leap. I have had two real flops in producing and marketing video reviews and some successes. Study the market carefully before producing a specialty product and be able to say "no" even if the people involved are very nice. Videos have a short shelf life and require constant updating. The capital demands are great.

Marketing, Marketing, Marketing. Marketing products and services is an enormous challenge. The number of times the phone rings is dependent on how many promotional pieces we have produced and the postal service has delivered. It is a constant challenge to determine which advertising medium is most effective. Promoters of one medium are absolutely certain that their method is most effective. The reality is no approach is as effective as heralded.

No one is indispensable. Since writing the original story I have had several office managers. When the second manager decided to leave and work closer to her home, I was very upset and wasted considerable time and energy worrying about replacing her. I was able to do so with someone who was absolutely fabulous.

Treat your help well. Treat an employee well and they will be loyal. Pay an honest wage and make the work environment as friendly and comfortable as you can.

Make lemonade out of lemons. Recently when an unexpected office manager vacancy occurred, I decided not to worry and to promote one of my daughters to the office manager position. Of course, this is the daughter who, during her high school years, complained the loudest about having to help Mom at the office. She is now extremely efficient and capable. Another example of the interesting circles in the journey we call life.

Ideas come from interesting places. I sold learning games in my bookstore. Nursing faculty were always asking me if I had games for fluid and electrolytes, acid-base and pharmacology calculations— all of the subjects faculty hate to teach and students hate to sit through. The games weren't available so I developed them. Producing and marketing learning games is a challenge. It is quite a leap from questions on index cards to a marketable game. Faculty frequently tell me, "I developed a game for class. I should have marketed it." Little do they know of the process involved in such an enterprise. So, I developed a workshop to teach game development to faculty. I am not worried about teaching myself out of game sales, quite the opposite.

Listen to the inner voice. I need to allow myself to grow and change. I still love to teach and am very good at it. I have recently developed a passion for holistic health and energy medicine. I am now pursuing advanced studies in this field and am anxious to do more work in this area. The call for hands on work is once again becoming clear. I am preparing to change my focus to do more holistic nursing and energy work. The seeds are planted and hopefully they will grow. Once again the circle of life manifests.

When you work for yourself you have the most difficult taskmaster of all. The hours are long, the work is hard, but the satisfaction is great. There are downs as well as ups but in the end it is well worth it. Occasionally I wonder what it would be like to know for certain how much money will be in my paycheck at the end of the week or what it would be like to have someone else write me checks on a regular basis or what it would be like to go home at the end of the day and forget about work. I wonder these things, but not for long. Because then I have another idea for a product or workshop I want to do.

Nursing Tutorial & Consulting Services
11804 Wolf Run Lane
Clifton, VA 20124
(800) US-TUTOR

Chapter 14

Reimbursement:
A Consultant's Focus

(This profile appeared in the November 1989 issue of the *Nurse-Entrepreneur's Exchange.*)

Editor's Note: GM Associates, a consulting firm providing expertise on a wide spectrum of healthcare issues, was founded by Glenda Motta, RN, MPH, ET, in 1987.

Through a combination of talents, the group offers healthcare industry clients a creative approach to disseminating ever-changing technical information using a wide variety of vehicles and methodologies.

NEE: What was your motivation to start GM Associates?
Glenda: "Running a home health agency for three years exposed me to the reimbursement end of things for the first time. This was back in 1975, and it was the first home health agency that was in competition with Visiting Nurse Associations. This was before for-profits could become Medicare certified.

After graduate school in 1980, I went into consulting and worked for a year on Health Care Finance Administration contracts. Then, for four years I worked for a consulting firm outside of Washington, D.C. This is where I developed the skills that I now have. And after progressing from manager to director, running a half-million dollars worth of contract work, and doing all the marketing, proposals, and reimbursement work; that is when I began to think about starting my own business.

I was then elected president of the International Association of Enterostomal Therapy, which required a lot of time, and the firm I was with was not supportive of my outside efforts. So I made the decision to break with them, accept the presidency, and start my business."

NEE: Where do your clients come from?
Glenda: "I had contact with a manufacturer—by virtue of being an ET nurse and being active in the Association, and had been talking with them for a year about a project at the company I was with. When I told them that it looked like I would be leaving, they said, 'We want to go with you.' So they became my first client, and within my first month I had a contract.

Since then, most of my clients have come from word-of-mouth. Also, I lecture at many places where industry is exhibiting. Now, for the first time, I'm actively marketing GM Associates by mailing out Corporate Capability packages."

NEE: Are reimbursement-related projects your primary focus?
Glenda: "Yes. If you look at our services—the economic studies, market research, publications, and newsletters—they're all geared in some way toward reimbursement.

My clients are mostly medical device manufacturers who come to me for a number of reasons. First, they may have an existing product that they're getting reports on of reimbursement problems. Or they need general education to understand the reimbursement climate of how their products fit into all the arenas, from acute care to skilled nursing care to home health, and how both federal and private insurance affects the use of their products.

94

If it's new product development, they come to me because many of them have been mandated to investigate the reimbursement climate prior to either acquiring new technology, or introducing new technology on the market. So they need to know how to price that technnology, and what they need to do to ensure that their product will be reimburseable."

NEE: What are the reimbursement options for medical devices?
Glenda: "Historically, insurers used to pay for everything without question. Now, Medicare can elect not to reimburse for technology if they believe it's experimental, so the onus is on the manufacturer to prove that it is acceptable medical practice. They also have to demonstrate medical necessity, safety and efficiacy, and cost-effectiveness."

NEE: What specific activities does GM Associates do?
Glenda: "We research and prepare the documentation necessary for a company to go to the insurer to educate them, and in Medicare's case, to obtain what's called an alpha-numeric code for the product. This identifying code number is required for the purpose of billing. The National Blue Cross Association has a Technical Review Panel that you make a presentation to, then they make a decision on whether to pay for the product. It is still so decentralized, Medicare included, that each carrier has the power to make their own decision on payment and coverage.

I'm also doing a lot of co-sponsored educational programs geared towards nurses in different settings. I lecture extensively on reimbursement and other related issues, such as how documentation is tied to payment, litigation, and quality."

NEE: What time frame do your projects take to complete?
Glenda: "It depends on the project. Most are done in two to three months, but I had another project that involved putting together a reimbursement manual for a sales force of 150 salesmen. The com-

ponents of that involved a lot of research, in terms of talking to fifty different Medicare carriers, and getting a questionnaire completed so that each one of these sales people had information specific to their locale. That project took a year to complete."

NEE: What's your advice to nurses wanting to go into business for themselves?
Glenda: "Network! If industry is your target, then get into a position where you can interact with industry on a professional level. Then, the business just grows out of that because of the credibility you've established."

GM Associates
11012 Childs Street
Silver Spring, MD 20901
(301) 593-6250

Chapter 15

Nurses:
An Unsophisticated Market?

by Lizabeth J. Augustine, RN, BSN

I can still remember walking out feeling angry. Depressed. Belittled.
I had gone to one of the major insurance companies for a sales position in response to an ad in *The New York Times*, and when asked
who I wanted to do business with I immediately replied, "nurses." I
was told by the interviewer that I would never make any money because nurses were an unsophisticated market.

I was reading his mind as I listened to him ramble on about the business of insurance and investment sales. He was visualizing nurses
with thermometers, bedpans, and maybe even IV's. He had no idea
what I was capable of doing based on my experience. He had no
idea about the power of nurses. I left his office with a real goal in
mind. Simply put, I knew someday I would prove him wrong.

It is with great pleasure that I find myself four years later in business
for myself as well as part of the Equitable Financial Companies Network, a company I'm proud to say shared my vision that nurses mat-
tered. In both facets of my business life I run seminars and individual consultations to tell nurses how to gain a more firm financial
footing. And even in these uncertain economic times my business is
booming.

I'd be lying if I said starting a business was easy. It's not. Far from it. Expect to shed a lot of sweat and a few—no, make that many—tears as well. But that old cliche about things worth having are worth fighting for is true. You've heard "no pain, no gain." Believe it. I'm not trying to sound discouraging—only truthful. Just don't put off that idea or goal. Start today. Start *now*. You too can have your own business. It's never too early to plan. And planning ahead now will make your path to both owning your business and financial independence that much smoother.

My own road was not always so smooth, and I offer this story in the hopes that you might benefit from knowing that you can make a difference in your own life. That part is the hardest. As nurses, we have been conditioned to always make a difference in others' lives, and we all have experienced phenomenal outcomes both on and off the job. It is time to turn that energy into yourself. As nurses, you know we have a lot in common. We're sensitive people, drawn to help others; we're tough and adaptable. These are strengths which can be used in the business world. If we draw on our common strengths, but add to that helping ourselves in addition to helping others, we are unstoppable.

It is important to share some of my personal background with you, because I believe that many of us have a tendency to think that it takes extra brains, extra money, or extra whatever to own your own business. Yet, it just takes extra guts—it is all up to you if you are willing to find out who you are, what you want and why you want it. I started out in a typical family; I was the oldest of three children and the only girl. We were close knit and loving. I'm sure that's where my maternal nurturing side comes from. If there was a downside to growing up in New York, it was that we were cash poor most of the time. You could describe us as lower middle class. I was a happy child who never wanted for anything— food, clothing, or shelter. But honestly, I grew up with a sense that the necessities could be taken away at any time. It may have been an irrational fear, but it's a vivid memory. I'm sure that is where the basis of both my selves came from. The nurturing side wants to take care of everyone, and the child who remembers never having enough money was determined that she should find ways to become financially independent.

My parents did teach us about hard work and how it could pay off. They also taught me to be goal-oriented. For that, and for all they did, I will always be grateful. My dad, in particular, told me that it would be in my best interest to always be solely responsible for supporting myself. This notion —that a man wouldn't be there to support me—was a radical notion in my family.

When I was in my late teens my family moved to upper middle-class suburbia. My mother's dream. And she taught me that dreams do come true. But talk about culture shock. I went from feeling that the necessities would go away to literally trying to keep up with the Joneses—it was strange to walk to school when so many kids were driving brand new cars. Their own cars no less. It would be an understatement to say it was a most confusing time. But I saw first-hand, as we went up the financial rungs, that money meant power, and power meant more freedom.

Education was also stressed by my parents. If you want something, go for it, they would say; but it helps to know what you are going for and how to go about getting it. By the time I decided to go to college I knew I wanted to be a doctor. I wasn't the typical little girl who wanted the nursing uniform, but realistically I knew that affording eight to ten years of higher education was out of the question. So I happily opted for nursing, knowing that I would still be helping people. I also knew that I would always be employed and make money.

Being a nurse came easy to me; there was something natural about it. It was in my blood. I saw people at their worst—complaining, in pain, helpless, arresting. Nothing bothered me. I even impressed myself with my ability to catch on so fast.

I began my nursing career in 1982. My first year and a half was spent in a tiny, sedate community hospital that ran smoothly and efficiently. Everyone should have a job experience like my first opportunity. As a person who always thrived on excitement and even a little stress, I decided to leave for a challenge of a larger, more rambling hospital in urban New York. More culture shock—but I'm used to that, remember?

My first assignment was in a neurology unit, a roach-laden neurology unit. It wasn't pretty. It was also understaffed, dirty, noisy, cramped. Get the picture? Imagine a *MASH* unit without the humor. Patients were desperately, terminally ill and nurses didn't have the times to share the simplest of courtesies with the grieving families.

I recall, hesitatingly, one especially dismal time—a rainy and cold weekend. I was at the nurse's station, personally assigned to sixteen patients. All their call lights were on at the same time, and the place was witnessing a chaos unusual even for a usually chaotic place. Fortunately, while I was attending to the patients, a light went off in my head, too. I knew this hospital needed some remedial fixing— badly. I had ideas. But I was "only" a nurse—and a nurse making less than $30,000 a year. Who would listen to me? I wanted to call the president of the hospital and say, "Come up here and look at this- would you want to be treated this way?" We all know, of course, that he would be treated as a VIP, so he'd never know the reality of the situation.

My parents had often talked about how money was power, and I realized for the first time that they were so right. It had sunk in. I had the ideas. The brains. And the drive. But one major ingredient was missing. The power to do anything about it. I also didn't have the financial resources to leave. For the first time in a long time in my life, I felt stuck. It's a horrible feeling. But what my parents had been telling me all those years finally hit home.

I was powerless as a nurse, but only because of my income and pecking order of hospital hierarchy. The thought also came to me that nurses needed to become financially aware and, ultimately, fiscally empowered. A radical idea. But not an insane one. Thus began the idea for providing financial services for nurses.

Meanwhile, my own self-esteem was being seriously challenged. I had always been a go-getter, and this hospital was so mired in problems that I somehow made myself responsible for many of the problems. If only I could work harder, I convinced myself many nights before collapsing after my shifts. I had no life. My life was spent trying to help others, and I wasn't even doing a very good job of helping myself. I was a classic burnout victim although I didn't know it at the time. I thought I could be "cured" with a vacation. All I needed was to get away for awhile. But running away never solved any problems. In fact, when I came back from a brief vacation, the problems were still there and looming extra large. I noticed my pearl white shoes and uniform were covered in stains—blood, iodine, worse. I looked like I'd been through a battle. Looking back, I guess in some ways I felt I *had* been through a war. The blood stains, which once didn't bother me, stained more than just my clothes. It seemed I never left the hospital, and when I did go home I took the job with me.

My attitude was in need of a complete overhaul. I had nothing left. Still, I did my job. And did it well by all accounts. But I worked without humor, compassion, love, caring or generosity. I wasn't a nurse really. I was a machine.

I contemplated going back to the cute little hospital in the leafy tree suburb, but I knew that wasn't the answer. I asked for a transfer to the Neonatal ICU. I figured that looking at babies all day—innocent babies so in need of help—would give me some much needed perspective. At the very least I figured I wouldn't sit around feeling sorry for myself. The wing was designed to handle about fifty babies; we routinely took on as many as eighty. Eight months of Neonatal ICU and I came to the end of my rope. So much for intentions...

In two short years I went from being this naive, happy-go-lucky nurse who felt she could conquer the world, to someone who was burned out, bitter, helpless and, I'll admit, angry about the whole thing. So in late 1985 I quit staff nursing—I decided I could no longer be a part of the "problem." I promised myself (and I am the type of person who always keeps her promises) that I could not return under such conditions.

I did have to support myself. I'm no lottery winner. I don't have a rich husband. I'm not the type to rob a bank. And nursing was all I knew. I found myself doing things I had not done in a long while—taking long walks, relaxing, exercising, meeting friends. Little stuff, but very important. And the little stuff also included leisure reading, such as reading the paper and keeping up with current events.

One day while reading *The New York Times* I came across an ad that said: "Looking for a college graduate seeking unlimited earning potential..." And I said to myself, "Well, that sure fits me." The ad turned out to be for a sales position at a major insurance company. That's where I met the man who did not believe in nurses. However, I did become licensed through this company to sell insurance. He said I would be selling insurance and investment products, but that I would be responsible for creating my own client roster. That's wherethe "unsophisticated market" came in. I knew I would not be doing business with a man or a company so narrow minded, so bigoted, and so wrong. My gut instincts—and my stubborn streak—told me I was still on the right path, the path to lead myself and other nurses to their true potential.

Unfortunately, I still needed a job, and righteousness doesn't pay bills. I wondered if all financial companies felt the same way . I was getting depressed until I realized that *somewhere, somebody* must share my vision. Maybe a former nurse had made it. Or maybe I would meet with a company that believed that tapping into the nursing market might be a good idea after all.

After a most promising interview with The Equitable Financial Companies, I was introduced to a former nurse who was now a registered representative for the Equitable. Yes! A kindred spirit. Someone to bounce my ideas off of. She became an almost instant buddy. I signed on with The Equitable Financial Companies in March of 1987. Almost immediately I met with receptive groups, and nurses signed on asking me to tell them what they needed to know about money, insurance, and investments. I no longer considered that I had a job. I had a career. I see a career as something that you have for a lifetime. Something to be proud of, something to take stock in.

Ironically, at the time I was feeling so good about starting out on my own and making a financial future for myself, my area manager asked me how much I had in savings in order to work out my own individual financial strategy. I lied and said I had $1,000. It was actually more like $995 less than that. Funny but true. But I knew if I told the truth I might be laughed out of the office. As it was, they thought $1,000 was pretty funny. They kindly didn't laugh at me, but that is not to say that the early going was easy. I didn't laugh much, either. The first fifteen months I was in business were horrible. Working in the hospital, the one with roaches, even started to look good to me in hindsight. I wondered if I had done the right thing. I almost went back.

As any self-employed person knows, you have to do everything yourself, at least in the beginning. You must teach yourself the business and do the business at the same time. I had to learn about insurance and investment products and sell them at the same time. In between all of this commotion I had to find bodies to do business with, or there was no business to do. Talk about stress! I was always physically and financially lagging behind and was never quite sure why.

Horrible! Even now, as I think back to my early business days, I can think of no other way to describe it. I can make fun of it now, but I used to call it my "personal exorcism." I didn't realize how my nursing career had affected me. To put it simply, I was still blaming myself for things out of my control, such as making little mistakes that any new business owner was capable of making. In short, I was being too hard on myself.

Then I learned to sit back and relax. To enjoy my new role. To appreciate the good things. I knew from nursing that I could be flexible, adaptable, and highly organized in a pinch. Not to mention the people skills—I could be friendly at the most stressing times. Nurses know that this is a gift. So I called upon my many nursing strengths to get me through some of the rough moments. That made all the difference. I started to flourish, and now I wasn't just following orders, I was giving them.

Some of the tough moments for me in getting started in business involved working to put the anger behind me. I was angry for not having been insightful enough to save money earlier. I was angry with my parents (so helpful in many ways) for not stressing the importance of having money work for you. And I was angry with the nursing profession for paying us less than we are worth, and worse, not giving us the impetus to learn about how to take what we earn and turn it into something we could retire with. For those of you interested in starting your own business, I heartily recommend getting over these feelings. Learn from them, but don't hold onto them. They will do nothing but hold you back.

Also, and this is vitally important, I urge you to save up before taking the plunge. Try to save a minimum of $10,000. Here's why: my first year in business I made $18,000 and supplemented my income with $6,000 from per diem nursing. I was working more than fifty hours a week and was exhausted all the time when it hit me—I would make more money from hospital nursing. Talk about depressing.

Then a whole new group of unplanned expenses cropped up...Constantly. Bills seemingly came from nowhere. Now, common sense says I should have planned better, but who knew? I didn't. I almost put myself in a hole that I couldn't climb out of. I now had to wear more expensive clothes— along with their dry cleaning expenses. No more uniforms. I was wining and dining clients, which cost a lot more than the hospital cafeteria! The phone bills tripled. I had out-of-pocket expenses for things like stationery, travel, and developing clients. You get the idea. By the end of the first year I owed $15,000—more than half of my income. I knew enough about the business world to know that you didn't want the end of the year to show a debit or deficit. I didn't need a business degree for that.

I figured it was time for a bold move. Even though I owed so much, I started paying *me* and investing in *myself.* I put aside a modest $50 a month just for me and my future. I practiced what I preached. My self-esteem soared. My purpose was becoming clearer each day. And slowly the debit started to become less and less. I could see a profit looming in the not-too-distant future.

As I near my fourth year in business, my debt stands at far less than $1,000, which is ironic since that figure represents my "almost" savings level. I also now invest $1,000 a month in my future. With this symbolic figure I can now laugh, because I know that the good times are ahead. I now have confidence in myself, and I haven't been wrong yet. I guess I am proof positive that even when it looks bleak, a firm belief in self can get you through just about anything. Like nursing, business is just a series of short-and long-term goals. The only difference is that in business the process seems to focus more on you, whereas in nursing the emphasis seems to be focusing on everyone else first. That change does take a little getting used to. But it can be done. It is a rewarding lesson to be learned. And you deserve it. You've worked hard to get here. You should work equally hard to get what you want in life.

In addition to my personal business of counseling nurses in money planning, I do similar work contractually. Finally, I am proud to announce that I have also recently incorporated a new business. The company is called Health and Wealth For Life, Inc. We provide insightful seminars for nurses to educate them in self-esteem, finances, and planning for their increasingly bright futures.

It is not easy to own your own business. The hardest part was learning to trust myself and my instincts. I have worked at it constantly. In part, I am working this hard to personally see to it that nurses take fewer lumps than I did in getting a business off the ground. The past four years I have worked six days a weeks, anywhere from fifty to seventy hours per week. I still find time in my schedule to do at least one day a week of hospital nursing. My friends and family think I am crazy. But it's not for the extra money; I know now that money was never the reason I got into nursing. Nursing does many things for me that money never could. But I also know that the money I make in business gives me something. A future and security. It also gives me that power I talked about earlier that might allow me to get some of the power nurses need to change the healthcare system. Wouldn't that be great! We can make the world a better place. If I didn't believe that, I wouldn't be focusing my business on nurses. I believe in us.

UPDATE 1997

It is with great pleasure that I have an opportunity to once again participate with The National Nurses in Business Association. This March of `97 I will be celebrating ten years in business. The last five have been dedicated to fine tuning my mission of providing financial services to healthcare professionals.

I spent most of the last five years marketing my services locally and studying for the completion of my financial designations. In short, I have experienced many successes and challenges but two things have remained unchanged: A belief in my own ability to succeed and a strong dedication to the nursing profession.

I will be completing one of my financial designations in January of `97. This will afford me with greater opportunities. My business is now more organized than it ever was before and I am looking forward to working with the NNBA. I will share with you all this one thought: Persistency and a belief in your own ability will triumph over all challenges.

I believe every nurse should pursue a business opportunity to learn the lessons that present themselves and experience the rewards of being responsible for your own destiny. "Nursing is the Art of What is Possible" and I look forward to the possibilities that will present themselves through the NNBA. A special thanks to Laura Gasparis Vonfrolio for the opportunity to be with you all again.

Lizabeth J. Augustine RN, BSN, LUTCF
1221 Avenue of The Americas, 32nd Floor
New York, NY 10020
212-719-8720

Chapter 16

The Evolving Dream

by Martha Jean Minniti, RN,BS, CCRN

In 1980, I was working as an agency nurse while going to school to complete my Bachelor's in Psychology and finish my pre-med requirements. I had basically had it with nursing; I wanted out. I wanted to be in a position where I could affect healthcare, be part of the decision making process, and be where I could really have a positive effect on patients. I didn't feel I could do that any more in nursing—although I loved being a nurse—so I set my sights on medical school.

While working as an agency nurse I started to notice a lot of things. In those days agencies didn't have a very good reputation, and I noticed that the hospitals never knew who they were going to get. They didn't know if it would be a qualified nurse who could do a balloon pump in critical care, or if it was somebody who couldn't even start an IV.

I kept observing and saying to myself there's got to be a better way. That's when the idea of nurses being independent hit me. I believed the employer model was too parental for professionals and undermined the capacity of the professional in subtle and not so subtle ways. I believed that nurses needed to do more—especially agency nurses—to affect their own reputation. So, I started forming the concept that the ideal agency would be a network of reliable professionals with good credentials and experience, and that the agency would be the broker, getting both the nurses and the hospital the best arrangement possible. The broker would get their fee from the hospital, but it would be less than the agencies of the day, which had quite a mark up. I also thought this "agency" could design itself to wipe out the problems that had been associated with agencies and agency nurses of the past, ie: replacement for call out, service objectives, and independent quality assurance.

I also started to examine the agency concept from the nurses side. I was a good nurse, a nurse the agency I worked for would send out to a hospital they wanted to impress. But they didn't think twice about giving a new recruit my shifts, and that was very frustrating. And, I found that agencies—in general—were run by business people. I wondered how it could be different with healthcare professionals running the business.

After contemplating all of this, I told my boyfriend, who I was living with(now my husband). I went on and on about my frustrations and ideas, and he said, "Marty, either do something about it or shut up." I thought: that's it, I am not going to say another word, and I *am* going to do something about this. So, I stopped talking to him and started testing my ideas with some nurses. One of the staff nurses from a university hospital at which I had worked said to me that she had heard about my idea, thought it was great, and that she would love to work with me. This same nurse told a friend of mine, who was the Medical Director for Critical Care. Both of them came to talk with me about my idea and supported it. After all, they desperately wanted good help.

It has always struck me that there was a sequence of events that got set up—some of which I was responsible for and some I wasn't—that brought my company into formation.

One day I came into work, and this same staff nurse told me she had mentioned my idea to the Vice President of Nursing, who was interested. I went to see the VP and told her I was going off to medical school in September, but wanted something for the spring and summer, and that I wanted to broker myself to her directly. Initially, she did what most VPs of Nursing would do: she tried to talk to me into coming on staff, or on pool. I told her no; I wanted to do this as an independant contractor to set myself up in business and have a tax deduction, and that I wanted to function much like an attending physician—who, as a professional, could come in, take care of patients and do it on a contract basis. She understood, and kind of liked the model, but she said, "Marty, I cannot deal with individuals; it is just too difficult for the system."

Being an intrapreneur herself, she told me to get ten nurses together and we would do a contract. That was the beginning of Skilled Nursing, Inc. (SNI). From there, I tried to set the company up as a collective. I thought that if we did it as a collective it would work better, and that I could still go to medical school.

However, I could not find people who wanted to invest time, energy or money. They wanted to work through the company, but they didn't want the on call or legal responsibilities. So, it boiled down to myself and two other interested people.

Those two people eventually did not work out either. One was already picking out the color of his Mercedes before he was doing the work, so he didn't last. The other one was more grounded and responsible. But she really wanted to do education and didn't want the part of front line entrepreneur, so she decided to return to teaching and pursue a PhD. So, it ended up in a short period of time that I became the person who was running the company.

The company took off quickly. Within the first three months, SNI was staffing three major hospitals in Philadelphia. I was enthused about the business. It was a natural for me, although I had no formal training. I was driven to succeed. I couldn't sleep. I was obsessed with making things work. I found someone to organize the office,

111

and brought in nurses and others to help run the business.

Meanwhile, I still thought I was going to be a doctor. However, almost from day one, when I got to medical school I found that I did not like it. I didn't like the structure or the aggrandizement of a physician. I loved the knowledge and the idea of managing patients. I wanted to get patients away from having the doctor make health care decisions. It just didn't fit. As a nurse, I taught people how to think and care for themselves.

I was getting more and more disheartened with medical school while taking tests and attending lectures. I also found myself with two notebooks: one for medical school and one for business, and I was continuously getting business ideas. After three months, I left school and totally immersed myself in SNI.

Skilled Nursing, Inc. became the leading agency in Philadelphia. We turned around the model of what it meant to be an agency nurse. We have drawn to us some of the most competent nurses in the city—nurses who want to play with a different model of nursing: that of being an independent contractor. This model has brought a lot of creativity and professionalism to nurses. Today, SNI is a $20 million company, and four more companies have been started.

In 1985, I started a home care company, and there again I will say that the universe brought us to home care. We were being asked at SNI to bring sick patients home. These were patients that the other home care companies couldn't handle: the trauma, ventilator, and complicated hospice patients. We had adults and kids at home on ventilators, with all of their IV, enteral therapies and social family needs. Because most of these patients were private or commericial pay, and we were not yet Medicare certified, I realized if we wanted to do home care, we needed to get into it right. So, we created a Medicare home care company and then a private home care company. Both have grown tremendously. We are now a leading provider of home care, doing more than 60,000 visits, dealing with both complicated and traditional patients.

I kept looking at the SNI model and thinking this is wonderful because the nurses like it, and the hospitals benefit from flexible staffing and competent nurses, but I wanted to be more involved. I wanted to make more of a difference in the way units are run, and healthcare in general. I kept thinking that there were businesses out there that contract manage everything from entire healthcare business sectors to ERs to labs to pharmacies, and why can't nursing do this? Why can't we contract out whole units and have them run as business and professional units? So I created a company called Facilities Management, Inc. (FMI).

FMI managed an eight-bed medical ICU for three years and managed a contract with the government for part of a unit, and started to look at practice units with mixes of employees and contract nurses with new management models. The structure is similar to a professional practice unit, with attending nurses coming in as part of the unit. FMI still has a long way to go, but that was the beginning of contracting out nursing units. Some day, I believe there is the potential to contract out the entire nursing department—and I believe that some vice presidents have the same idea.

Then I had a nurse from Australia come talk to me who had been a foreign nurse. She felt there were a lot of good foreign nurses who wanted to come to the United States, but were dumped into situations that were not wonderful, professionally or personally. I agreed, and that became SNI USA, a company that brings foreign nurses to other countries—including the U.S.—and eventually became a specialty traveling nurse company in the United States.

Next on the drawing board is an IV and case management company. It fits with home care, so we are jumping in. We are also looking at going public.

To this day, I am amazed things happen that you want to happen—maybe not on your timetable—but when you have the intent, it *does* happen. I have learned much about running a company, an organization, and multiple companies.

I have also learned a lot about other nurse entrepreneurs. I speak about nurse entrepreneurship, and last year I sent out a questionnaire to nurse entrepreneurs and found that we are different. We are not just entrepreneurs; we *care* about our product immensely. We're involved in life enhancing work, quality of life improvement, and nurse empowerment. I am enthralled with the opportunities that are available to nurses today.

Today, there are more than 1,500 people who have brought their vision to The SNI Companies and have taken The SNI Companies vision to nurses. Together, our dreams and realities are taking form and coming true, and they are having a direct effect on improving options for nurses, patients, and healthcare.

Martha J. Minniti, RN, BS, CCRN
President/CEO
The SNI Companies
1811 Bethlehem Pike, Suite 112
Flourtown, PA 19031
(215) 836-9000

Chapter 17

A Day at the White House

by Angela Franklin, RN

It was May of 1988, and one of those rare, perfect days in Washington, D.C. Clear blue skies and soft gentle breezes. Almost serene. However, the tranquility was broken by the clicking of camera shutters, the echoes of microphones, and the chatter of reporters.

The chairs were arranged neatly in a "V" so that attention focused on the honorable speakers in front of us. I was seated in the Rose Garden of the White House among a collection of people from different states, all being recognized by the Small Business Administration for Small Business Person of the Year. We also joined together for the last step of the competition to await final acclaimation for the National Small Business Award of 1988, as only one company would claim that title.

The judgment process required much introspection and an in-depth analysis of my business. To substantiate meeting the strigent criteria in the areas of creativity, financial stability, management style, growth in personnel, and the ability to overcome adversity, we had to submit three-year financial statements, reference letters, a business autobiography, and a company video.

For me, this was the pinnacle of many years of hard work, dedication, and effort. I refocused my attention on the two speakers in front of me, President Reagan and Vice President George Bush. As

I listened to their views on the future of small business, I couldn't help but reflect on the past developments that had brought me to this point in my professional and business career as a nurse entrepreneur.

The decision to ultimately start this journey came as a result of trying to be a single parent with sole responsibility of support. Being a fresh nursing graduate in 1975, and raising a two-year old son myself, I worked graveyard shifts in the hospital so that I could sleep while he went to day care. Deciding the night shift created an imbalance in my biological clock, I went to evenings as an IV nurse. This didn't work because I had to rely on sitters, so I searched out the job market and hit the big one! Monday through Friday, 7a.m. to 3 p.m. on the IV team at a large teaching hospital in Los Angeles.

I thought I was finally set, until a phone call came early one morning just before I was paged to go the Respiratory Intensive Care Unit. My sitter called to say that she would be leaving my son alone because she'd missed his day care bus and she had to go to school. I put the call behind me and rushed to the unit. I tried to find a vein to insert the angiocath into my patient, while my mind was several miles away on my two-year old that would be left alone—possibly all day. My train of thought was broken as a co-worker tapped me on the shoulder to explain that my patient had expired before I arrived. Oh, God! How embarrassing! I didn't even notice that there were no vital signs, let alone veins. That was it—I combed the newspapers for something that would give me more flexibility and independence, and there it was—home healthcare, the beginning!

I worked for three fledgling companies in Los Angeles, and learned as much as I could possibly absorb. This finally afforded me the flexibility I had been looking for, but I still did not have the financial independence and control of my destiny that I wanted. A co-worker friend always reminded me that I had told her that at this time next year, I would have my own company making $50,000 a year. At the time, I didn't know how or where I would do this.

A year later I moved to Northern California. I worked for a few months as a nursing supervisor for a new private home health company in Stockton. That's where I met my soon-to-be business partner, who was by trade a social worker transplanted from Florida. We worked diligently for this company, and developed everything from marketing strategies to clinical systems and business forms. Our office grew to be the most productive in the Western Region. One day, I had to research some information, and no one in the company—not even on the regional or national level—would help. I realized that the time had come to do all of this for myself.

My co-worker also recognized the abilities that we possessed, and readily accepted the opportunity to have a business of our own. We had signed a two-year non-compete agreement with the company we had just left, and so, to honor this, we ventured down the highway to a town colled Modesto in Central California. I had no idea where Modesto was, but I knew that I had something to offer it.

We brainstormed together. I wanted *PRN* in our company name to designate a service that would be there when needed. Then, I built a name around it: Professional Reliable Nursing. We incorporated in June of 1979. We now had an identity, and so played with designing a logo that would give us quick recognition

We finally gave birth to the company, but now had to find the means to support it. We put together a list of all expenses—relying on experience from past operations—and developed a budget to use for obtaining capital funding. We then approached a newly developed local bank to ask for a $15,000 loan. This would be the beginning of our banking relationship. We met with the bank president, and presented our budget and our collateral: a 1936 Pontiac and a silver set.

In, retrospect, we must have received our granted loan of $9,000 on blind enthusiasm and proven hard work ethics, because they accepted neither the Pontiac nor the silver set for collateral. We also completely omitted all payroll taxes and obligations from our budget, and, being in a labor intensive business, that was a large part of our expenses. These were hidden administrative costs that I did not think of when I was on the employee end of the employer/employee relationship.

We already had the forms and systems that we had previously developed , a $9000 loan, a company identity, and a geographic market area. But how was anybody to know we were there? We solved this dilemma by flipping through the Yellow Pages in a phone booth, and permanently borrowed the pages with the headings: *Physicians, Social Services, Nurses,* and *Hospitals*. This became the basis for a marketing plan and competitive analysis.

We rented a tiny office, bought desks and business forms, designed a brochure, and advertised for nurses who wanted to work in the home care field. Our first week we earned $90. We worked every aspect, including scheduling, marketing, bookkeeping and janitorial.

We made presentations everywhere: service clubs, pharmacies, doctor's offices, senior groups, retirement centers, and anybody else who would listen to us. By the end of 1982, we had built a stong clientele.

We had initially started out to provide home care, but we received so many calls from hospitals for supplemental staffing, that in the first six months of operation only 5 percent of our work was home care. The company made the $50,000 that I had proclaimed the previous year. But a boycott by the hospitals on our supplemental staffing services left us scrambling to focus on providing the service that we had initially intended to provide—home care.

We quickly created an intense promotion for home care using the large pool of nurses that we had, and managed to capture our market niche within a few months. We almost *asked* for the most difficult of patient situations, for that gave us the reputation as an innovative company and a strong patient advocate. We worked with the California Department of Health Services to develop the Medi-Cal ventilator-dependent home care program, and also the first congregate living situation.

Today, PRN Services, Inc. focuses on providing home healthcare services to all age groups. The corporate office is in Modesto, with a branch established in Stockton in 1981. Our service area is five counties, including San Joaquin, Stanislaus, Calaveras, Tuolumne, and South Sacramento. We provide skilled services of RN's, LVN's, home-health aides, nurse's aides, live-in companions, and housekeepers. Specialized care includes pediatrics, IV therapy, ventilator-dependent and hospice support.

We now distribute approximately 300 employee checks every two weeks. This year, sales will approach $3.5 million. I credit this largely to good systems and a strong management style. I have always believed in empowering my employees in a team environment. I believe that all employees contibute collectively towards the goals of the company, and should be rewarded equally. They are responsible for program development, annual goals, budgets, and their own reward system.

It is this approach that has allowed myself and my partner to move on to additional ventures. She has now married, inherited four children, and has since moved to Colorado. And I have developed A.K. Franklin & Associates. As a consulting company I have assisted other businesses—both home health and non-medical—in market development, competitive analysis, and strategic planning. I have also positioned myself in what I believe is an up-and-coming field in long-term care as a case manager performing assessments for insurance companies. I still volunteer much time in an advisory capacity as a board member to the California Association for Health Services at Home, a mentor through the Small Business Administration, and as an advisor to long-term care facilities.

I have developed throughout the years some hard-fast rules that I operate by, and I truly gained them by graduating from the school of hard knocks and experience, since neither my partner nor I had any business background. The first thing that kept me focused is what I call my *anchor*. This is the reason(s) that you are in business. For business is never smooth sailing, and you will need to rely on your anchor to keep you focused thourgh the tough times. For me, it was having the capability of being financially independent, and being able to see my son grow up with some semblance of a normal home life.

In running a company, it helps to have a first-hand working knowledge of all areas of the business. This makes it easier to train additional staff as you grow. Identify potential problems fast and cut down on the need for additional capital.

Develop what you consider to be your niche, and also your "basics." We focused on home care. Being locally owned made it easier and quicker to respond to community and consumer demands. Our basics were solid direct-sales relationships using presentations, volunteering time, assisting in fund raising, and taking on challenging patient situations. Whenever we feel that we are scattering our efforts, our employees refocus on the basics—those fundamental strategies that got us moving in the beginning.

Seek out and maintain good professional help and support. I cannot express the importance of a good banking relationship, an accountant, and an attorney. You will draw upon their advice constantly throughout your business. My first attorney advised my partner and I that the biggest challenge would not necessarily be the business, so much as it would be the partnership. It is, as he proclaimed, "truly a marriage."

Realize that an opportunity might not always remain positive, and be willing to recognize it. I can count several patients who, in the beginning, were prime cases that presented a challenge and a good profit. But sometimes the scale tips and the challenge outweighs the profit. Knowing how much time (which equals dollars) goes into this challenge might just have you come up in the negative. Be willing to cut it loose!

Develop a master plan, and revise it whenever you need to. I didn't have a written business plan or market plan upon development of the company. But all the pieces were informally in practice. A written plan keeps you on track as you grow, and also lets everyone in the company know where they fit into the goals. Have written policies and procedures in place. You may need to draw upon them to save yourself in a labor dispute, and, on the positive side, employees want to know what is expected of them and how they are doing.

Quality brings quantity. Consumer psychology shows that people will pay more if they perceive that they are getting more. Don't be afraid to charge for a quality service, and, on the flip side, be willing to provide services at a discount, particularly when you "pioneer" a program.

Finally, seize the opportunity to let the public know how great you are. Public relations is the least expensive and most productive form of advertising. Whenver you do something great or challenging, write a press release. Develop a relationship with the editors of your newspapers or trade journals, and keep your name and company in their forethoughts.

There are five lessons that I have learned—they stand out in my mind because they are always those stumbling blocks that put you back ten steps to go ahead two. One, seek out good professional help and advice from the beginning, even if you think you can't afford it. Our first bookkeeping "system" was developed on a steno pad. This was not a sound foundation—had we spent a little extra money on a good system and some advice, it would have saved time and money. Find a good accountant, and develop a financial system that fits your company—and grow with it. Knowing where you are financially at all times is the fine line between making and breaking you.

Two, develop budgets and stick to them. I've made a lot of money, and let some of it slip through our fingers because we didn't stick to a budget. It's too easy to think that you'll always have excess cash, but sometimes you will need those extra dollars to fund your company growth.

Third, diversify your marketplace. Never count on business from one source. Twice throughout my business career, I had to "fall back and punt." Once in the beginning, when we had to refocus on home care services, and then later on when the insurance industry tightened reimbursement standards. I learned then to maintain a mix of revenue sources from both private and third-party insurance.

Fouth, employers and employees outgrow each other. There's nothing more painful than seeing a devoted employee unable to grow with the company. Or, a good employee that professionally grows faster than the company. It was a tough emotional lesson to realize this does happen in business, and that it's okay.

Fifth, roadblocks and failures are truly an opportunity to try a different approach to the same problem or situation. To me, this is what teaches you to be quick on your feet, and approach business on an instinctual level.

Professional Reliable Nursing Service, Inc.
1545 St. Marks Plaza, Suite 1-A
Stockton, CA 95207
(209) 474-1006

Chapter 18

Built On Quality: Committed To Service

(This profile appeared in the November 1988 issue of the *Nurse Entrepreneur's Exchange.*)

Editor's Note: In 1982, Elizabeth (Libby) Dayani, RNC, MSN, co-founded American Nursing Resources, Inc. (ANR) with her husband John Dayani, PhD. With corporate offices in Overland Park, Kansas, ANR provides supplemental staffing and home care nationwide through twenty-four offices in eleven states.

*Sales in 1982 were $772,000, and in 1986 were more than $15 million, which placed ANR 118th on **Inc. Magazine**'s 1987 list of the 500 fastest-growing private companies in America.*

Dayani's background includes becoming an family nurse practitioner in 1972, running a pediatric clinic in a housing project, teaching in an FNP program, and working for a public health department setting up a network of clinics.

NEE: What motivated your extensive background as a nurse practitioner?
Libby: "I have enjoyed the nurse practitioner role because I grew up in South America—my parents were missionaries, and I wanted to go back and run a clinic in the jungles of Brazil. I lived down there until I was thirteen, and my image of nursing from the beginning has

been colored by that experience. I imaged myself from the time I felt God had called me to be a nurse at age eleven, as an autonomous and respected practitioner.

You see, the only time I saw a doctor was once a month, when he'd come by in a jeep to do surgery. So I saw nurses doing the primary care—I didn't have to experience role re-socialization. If anything, I had to adapt to the way nurses were treated in America. The first time a doctor yelled at me I thought, 'Hey, this doesn't fit with my self-image as a nurse—he's not treating me with respect, what's his problem?' So I came into nursing with a clear image of what I saw nursing's potential to be. That's why, in my career, I have always looked for—and developed—roles for nurses that allow a great deal of autonomy and control over their practice."

NEE: What is the story behind ANR's origin?
Libby: "In 1977, we moved to Kansas City, and John went to work for his brother, who had founded Kimberly Nurses. John worked as vice president and learned the business side, and for the next five years I taught at the Kansas University School of Nursing. In 1982 John's brother died, and Kimberly was sold. John received an inheritance, and with part of it bought a company called Medifax. We founded ANR with the remaining money, and have continued to grow and learn ever since.

We now have offices in twenty-four cities, and people ask us, 'How do you decide where to go?' The answer is that we go where we find people. We don't say, 'Okay, these are the top ten cities in the U.S.— we're going to run ads and open offices.' We are not interested in being the largest in terms of offices; we go after people. If you've got the right person, every city is a marketplace."

NEE: What services did ANR provide initially?
Libby: "Back in 1982 we did supplemental staffing, although the nursing shortage that had been so critical in '79 and '80 came to a

screeching halt. When I opened this office, it was depressing because nobody needed supplemental staffing.

Fortunately, because of my background, I moved us into home care right away. We opened five offices doing private-pay home care and Medicare, and formed a second corporation called ANR Home Health Agency, Inc. In May of 1982, we Medicare-certified Memphis, St. Louis, Kansas City, and Austin. That was still a good time to get into Medicare, because now we tell our offices they cannot diversify into Medicare unless they can develop a joint venture with a hospital or physician group.

So, the bulk of our business in the early days was in home care; now it's about 50-50. But no two offices are alike. We have offices that do 100 percent home care, and a couple of offices that do 100 percent supplemental staffing.

We don't try to make our offices alike, because we believe that the office is built around the strength of the nurse executive and the needs of the marketplace. For example, our Phoenix office initially did primarily pediatric home care because that director's skills were in pediatrics.

We also encourage our people to diversify when they can, because of the safety in diversification. Any office that's doing primary supplemental staffing right now had better start thinking about home care, because I believe that the nursing shortage cycle is going to end in a couple of years. As hospitals develop different staffing patterns, they'll decrease their need for nursing, which will decrease the need for supplemental staffing. When that happens, we hope our office is already in home care so that the volume will grow in that area.

Our Kansas City office is our largest and most diversified because John and I believe we need to be hands-on managers; we need to demonstrate different models and business lines. We feel we don't have a right to say to our nurse executives, 'Go diversify and you figure out how to do it.' We try as many different marketing plans, joint ventures and ideas as we can come up with. And as we are successful in them, we are available to teach our nurse executives how to do it.

On the other hand, some of our offices have developed programs that all of us have benefited from. For example, the Phoenix office developed the pediatric protocol for home care. Rather than reinventing that in every office, we make that available to everybody through the corporate office, and if people want to call or visit each other for hands-on experience, they can do that. So it's a network of expertise that we make available to one another."

NEE: What is the greatest challenge you face in running a large corporation?
Libby: "Turning nurses into executives. Because nurses do not have a background. We haven't been taught how to think about numbers and marketing."

NEE: How do you teach business savvy to your people?
Libby: "Initially, we did it by having frequent telephone contact. John handles the business side, and I mentor the nursing and quality issues. He probably spoke to each office and every director at least once a week during the couple of years when we weren't so large. That probably had more to do with our success than anything, because John is very dynamic and motivating.

Then we went through a period when we didn't have as much time to spend talking with people as they needed, so we've implemented what we call Corporate Liaisons. We care about our people; we want people to learn how to succeed. And that happens through a lot of dialogue. So our Liaisons travel frequently to our offices to sit down and say, 'Okay, what's going on, why is this working and this not working; where do you think we ought to diversify?'"

NEE: Who oversees the finances of your individual offices?
Libby: "We have a Director of Finance at the corporate office that works with the nurse executive to develop a budget. There is not a wonderful margin in the business, so we work carefully with people to decide when they need to add staff and what amount of revenue is needed to pay for that staff."

NEE: How does ANR motivate and reward its people for success?
Libby: "The nurse executives receive stock after being with the company for eighteen months, and receive additional stock based on performance. We have a base salary with profit sharing, also based on performance. You need multiple incentives, because you can potentially have a volume of $1 million or more, and not be profitable. Generally, the profit margin in this business runs 1-3 percent, compared to 10-20 percent for medical equipment."

*NEE: In 1982, you co-authored **The Nurse Entrepreneur**. How did that project come about?*
Libby: "In 1981, I was trying to decide whether to get a PhD or write a book, and I decided to do the book. Because I'd always been interested in autonomy for nurses, I realized that business was one way that nurses could gain control over their practice. As a business person, you have greater control over defining the type of service you do in the hospital setting."

NEE: ANR recently bought Nurse America, Inc., a traveling nurse company. How's it doing?
Libby: "It's really taken off. Part of it is better management and being in the right place at the right time. Also, nurses are really looking to travel. Maybe it's because nurses are getting more confident, and the salaries they're finally getting are allowing them to have more fun. At any rate, we've jumped from fifty nurses applying each month to around 300."

NEE: We feel more nurses will soon be independently contracting nursing services to facilities. What do you think?

Libby: "I hope to see that happen in the next six to twelve months. The time to do it is now. Say to the hospital, 'Tell us what your budget is; we can do it for 5-10 percent less and relieve you of the headaches.'

The future of healthcare reimbursement is going to revolve around the shared-risk concept. The appeal to the hospital has either got to be that you can do it for less, or that you share in the profit/loss risk. But to negotiate such a contract, nurses need to get some business savvy and know where the administrators are coming from. They need to learn how to develop a budget, and learn how to talk to a banker, lawyer, and accountant. Learn to be comfortable with the players. Because once you develop that expertise, it's a level playing field. Then you can negotiate with CEO's. It doesn't take a great deal of business expertise, but it does take some.

We need to be reading business literature, *Modern Health Care* and non-nursing journals, so we can see the bigger picture. We have to broaden our vision beyond nursing in order to do the best for nursing."

NEE: What is the essence of ANR's success?

Libby: "We put a lot of trust in our nurse executives. We interview these people thoroughly before we hire them to make sure that their philosophy is similar to ours, and our philosophy is service first— service and caring.

We at the corporate office are going to service the branch office, the nurse executive, and her staff. And it's their responsibility to service their direct care-givers and clients. From the top level down, that's our greatest strength—our commitment to service and caring."

American Nursing Resources, Inc.
11050 Roe Blvd., Suite 101
Overland Park, KS 66211
(800) 333-3369

Chapter 19

Could It Work Here?

by Carolyn Bruce, MSA, RN

My husband and I were spending a weekend in my home town of North Vernon, Indiana, visiting with relatives. At the dinner table I was, as usual, expounding to everyone about the activities of Lincolnland Visiting Nurse Association, Inc., where I was employed as the Executive Director—and loving every minute of it.

My brother-in-law said to me, "Why wouldn't something like that (home healthcare) work here in Jennings County?" In a casual manner I said, "Oh it probably would." He said, "Could you start an agency here?"

I replied, "I suppose I could, but you would have to find me a super nurse who was willing to learn the business." He said, "I've got one. She is tired of the traditional hospital nursing work and the ongoing battles and would like to do something else. She has a degree and several years experience in patient care and supervision."

Driving home later, I reflected on this conversation again and again, the wheels in my head turning almost as fast as those under the car. Could I? Should I? Would I? And *why*?

I was perfectly satisfied and happy in my present position, with a great deal of autonomy to manage our nonprofit VNA in the way that I thought it should be done. A good relationship with my board of directors, good staff retention, increasing volume of business producing increased revenues, costs under control, image of the company and the reputation of patient care was above par, a successful marketing program underway, and enough challenges and opportunities to keep me busy at least sixty hours a week. Who needs any more?

On the personal side—a good marriage to a physician radiologist and a beautiful home; the children were grown and on their own. My life was certainly not dull; there were more things to do than I had time for, and heavens, my income was not even needed for our lifestyle. How lucky I was! What else could anyone want?

Yet, that idea kept niggling at me for days. I wondered if I could do it. I had some vacation time available. Maybe I'd just jot some things down on paper that would have to be done: It would be 180 miles from here in another state—no competition or conflict there to Lincolnland. I'd need to get state guidelines for home health licensure, and if the right nurse was available, my sister had a business administration degree and was looking at job possibilities now that her children were approaching high school age.

About two weeks later, I called my brother-in-law. He just happened to be vice president of commercial loans in the local bank. "If I would pursue this idea, would you help finance the company?" He said, "Sure, tell me what you need."

My husband was not all that amicable and ready to agree. He did not understand why I wanted to take on more work. He had some objections to investing money with the risks involved and a questionable return. But he admitted that I had been quite successful with the nonprofit company. He also knew that I could be very persistent. My decision was to use money from refinancing some property that I owned in Indiana prior to our marriage and borrow the rest. That would not risk any of our joint investments. If I failed, I alone would lose.

My business plans included some notes on paper and a lot of things to do coursing through my mind. Had I not had an in-route to the banker who knew something about the home care business from listening to me in earlier family conversations, I would have had to be more precise in details.

I met *the* nurse, Dona Thomas, on a prearranged evening in a motel halfway between her home and mine. We talked for almost four hours. This was November of 1982, and it was almost as cold in the room as it was outside. Not a comfortable environment. Nevertheless, she was excited about the new venture. Given some time to think about it, she called within the week and said, "Yes, I'll do it."

I had neglected to discuss the actual operating management that would be needed and had presumed that my sister Vivian would carry this responsibility. I called to tell her that Dona had said yes, and I was ready to go with the idea. In a crushed voice she said, "Aren't I going to have anything to do with it?" Hurriedly I explained that yes, there was a big job for her which I had just assumed she understood. I had talked so much about the critical role of the nursing director that I had failed to describe the very important function of the business manager, which I was counting on her to do.

My preliminary work was done on evenings and weekends, both writing policy and giving directions on the telephone between my home in Mattoon, Illinois, and North Vernon. Vivian and I met at an outlet office furniture store and purchased the barest of necessities. She located office space and initiated employee recruitment with Dona's input to clinical staff. A local attorney was consulted to put together the corporate organization.

Within six weeks we were ready to open. I took a week's vacation from the VNA and went on-site for some fast and furious directing and instructing.

The thrill that I will always remember was when I walked into the new office at 7:45 a.m. on opening day, January 9,1983, and the phone was ringing from a lady who needed home health care. Dona and I made the first home visit, and we were off and running with the Jennings Visiting Nurse Association, Inc., a proprietary organization with a community nursing mission in an area that did not know about home healthcare. And I was the sole shareholder!

In 1990, that agency serves seven counties, has four offices and approximately sixty employees. I haven't made any money, but the company has some retained earnings, and I am very proud.

The reasonable success of that agency prefaced my decision to accept another challenge in 1985, when I purchased a home health agency in Granite City, Illinois, now known as Vaughn Home Health Care, for $1,000. The proprietor, who had established the business in 1983, had ceased operations, transferred all the patients, and terminated all staff. The only things left were some odds and ends of office equipment, all her records, *and*, her Medicare provider number and state license to operate!

That agency has been, and is now, about 50 percent private care. I knew there was profit potential if managed right. Four offices now serve several Illinois counties bordering St. Louis. That $1,000 investment, plus much hard work, again at night and weekends, has grown 5,000 percent in five years. Obviously, I have full administrative and clinical staff in that agency, also. My husband is a shareholder and serves on the governing board.

My full-time responsibility continued at the nonprofit organization which is now a multi-corporate, multi-million dollar enterprise serving eleven counties in East Central Illinois. No, I did not neglect this business. Yes, I am a workaholic.

From childhood I was taught that hard work was a way of life, and I wanted to be a nurse since I can't even remember. But then I learned that as a professional nurse, there were avenues available in the traditional business world if one wanted to pursue them. I also felt it necessary to be better academically prepared. Through this same period of time, I started and completed my master's degree in Health Administration. I had rich resources of experience to write many of the required papers. My work in healthcare is my vocation, avocation, and sometimes I consider it my recreation.

Much of the credit goes to the fine staff that I have worked with from long distance. Their dedication to manage the companies successfully is greatly appreciated. Many times they have to wait for me for an answer to an issue. But these managers also realize that they have opportunities for intrapreneurship, and they accept their responsibilities well.

Have I had down times? You are so right! Problems such as additional financing needed, cash flow, retention of staff, ups and downs in volume of business, and a difference of opinion with the Internal Revenue Service have all come up. I am one who thrives on stress, and I have a lot of energy. Much credit goes to my husband, who is non demanding and tolerant of my many hours spent in one office or another. I am glad I took the plunge.

Although I have served as a consultant to both of my companies for the past several years, I am now establishing a formal consulting business with the approval of my board of directors and will share my knowledge of the home health business and other services to a broader market.

From a unique view, I was not aware of all the efforts being made in the past few years to encourage nurse entrepreneurship until I attended the NNBA Nurse Empowerment conference in San Francisco in

May of 1990.

I had not realized until then that I was a nurse entrepreneur.

Associated Nurse Consultants
115 Doral Court
Mattoon, IL 61938
(217) 234-4044

Chapter 20

Going For Broke

by Jerry W. Chevalier, RN,MSN,CNS

Nursing has evolved and is still evolving from the subservient to the self-sufficient, branching out from typical bedside care to areas previously unheard of. Demand for higher accountability by professionals and public alike has opened opportunities for which the nurse is uniquely qualified. Where there is demand, there is a potential for profit, and where there is profit, there are risks as well as rewards.

The following passages describe how and why I started my business with tips and lessons I learned along the way. If any one theme can be extracted from my story, it should be one of *perseverance.*

When I was growing up, I enjoyed shows like *Perry Mason, Adam-12,* and *Emergency.* The ideal of helping the defenseless, wrongly accused, and the sick and injured appealed to me—probably because I had been abused and mistreated by others in the past. I intensely dislike those who prey upon or take advantage of others, but I also enjoy helping those in need. After some debate, I decided to become a nurse. However, after seven years of increasing responsibilities and duties without adequate financial compensation, challenge, or recognition (abuse of another form), it was beginning to take its toll on me and my satisfaction with hospital-based nursing.

Higher patient acuities, fewer nurses, low pay, and no respect from hospital administration contributed to my dissatisfaction, so I decided to explore other avenues. In the back of my mind I knew that there would be a time when I would somehow have to go out on my own. I was not happy working for somebody else.

I needed more autonomy and freedom than traditional nursing would offer. I wanted to utilize my existing knowledge and experience, but in a different arena, so I tried my hand at reviewing medical cases for attorneys on an independent basis. I found the investigative procedure and nature of the cases fascinating, and I wanted to do and learn more. As a consultant, my observations, knowledge, and experience counted for something. I started attending seminars and inservices and read numerous books and magazines covering an array of medical, legal, and ethical subject matter. I previewed instructional legal vignettes and attended mock trials as well as actual malpractice proceedings.

I believe that money, or the lack of it, is the primary reason why people do not go into business for themselves. I believe that anyone with determination who believes in her or his own ability and faith in the enterprise can be successful. It will not happen in a week or a month form now, but it will happen.

I had to start my business on a shoestring—lean and mean with not much in between. I did not have the luxury of resource capital or the ability to get a business loan, so I had to work as an agency nurse while I was developing my business. I simply could not afford to make mistakes, and I think it was that which made me work harder and smarter.

In my office, I have two posters prominently displayed. They represent my philosophy of a business and how I started. The contents of one of the posters is known by just about every nurse. It reads: *We the willing, led by the unsure, are doing the impossible for the ungrateful. We have done so much for so long with so little we are now qualified to do anything with nothing.* The other poster is less familiar to nurses, but it describes what happens to most businesses when they start to become complacent. It reads: *Upon the plains of hesitation lie the blackened bones of countless millions, who, at the dawn of victory, sat down to rest, and resting, died.*

I started my business with no resource capital. Fortunately, I already had the three most important items needed to start up a consulting business: the belief in what I was doing, the drive to make it so, and a computer system. Most any computer with a decent work processor, database package, and a letter-quality printer would do.

However, I am what is known in the computer industry as a *power user*. I like technology, and I make it work to my advantage. My wife and I have accumulated an impressive computer system which consists of a Tandy 4000, an 80386 computer with 16 megabytes of extended memory, two high capacity disk drives, an Intel math coprocessor; a Seiko Instruments CM-1440 Super VGA monitor (1024x768) for high resolution graphic printing and professional looking documents; a US Robotics 2400 baud internal modem; a Niscan GS hand scanner; a Colorado 60 Mb external tape backup unit; and an Ilitachi 1503S external CD-ROM drive to access massive amounts of data and information.

All of my software is Microsoft Windows oriented. We use Word for Windows, a powerful graphic oriented word processing package; Microsoft Excel for spreadsheet and accounting activity (better than Lotus 1-2-3); Superbase 4, a powerful relational database package; Crosstalk for Windows for telecommunications to national database information services; and PageMaker for graphic intensive publication development for illustrative reports, manuals, brochures, etc.

This equipment and software is not cheap, and it took many hours to learn and understand so that it could be utilized efficiently and effectively. Whatever system you use, make sure that it will do what you want it to do, and that you can get support from your dealer (I would be happy to help you pick the kind of system for your business). Now, this is by no means a requirement for a successful business, but it sure helps!

With my equipment, I developed my business and Rolodex cards, letterhead, the art work, layout, and logo for my brochure. I obtained letters of reference from my clients and used them as testimonials to solicit additional business. I obtained referrals from my existing clients, from mailing lists of attorney-oriented magazine companies, the public library, and the yellow pages. Using my computer, I located and placed notices on free, attorney-oriented computer bulletin boards. Since my business is a non-testifying, professional consulting expert service, it is generally acceptable to advertise. So I placed ads in law-oriented magazines and had a yellow page listing.

Generally, I would try to get an appointment with the attorney who deals with malpractice or product liability cases. However, that is not always possible. Attorneys are crisis oriented. Consequently, they do not have much time to waste. That is why they have their secretaries screen calls, and this can be a problem if you cannot get through the front door. One technique is to have the name of the person or firm that referred you and tell the secretary something like this: "Hello, I am (your name). I need to speak to (name of attorney) about a malpractice case. I was referred by (name of referring attorney or other contact)." This way you do not reveal your true reason for the call, which is to solicit business. If the attorney is too busy or simply unavailable, then call him back (up to three times). If he does not return your calls, then send your service information packet and follow up again in a few days. Our packet consists of a cover letter, brochure, promotional pen, five business cards, two Rolodex cards, resume, letters of reference, and a sample report. Then periodically, I would send updates on any new services or available inservices.

My firm is called MedLaw: Medical Litigation Consultants. MedLaw is a professional consulting expert service designed to assist the plaintiff or defense attorney in the evaluation of delivered healthcare. We provide a comprehensive and cost-effective service consisting of medical record reviews for merit, inservices, client interviews, medication analysis, query assistance before and during deposition and trial proceedings, medical information research and procurement, expert witness preparation which includes practical and videotaped examples outlining proper conduct, dress and body language; how a witness should and should not answer questions; and tricks, traps, and techniques employed against the witness. A "day in the life..." video graphically depicting the impact of a disability and the difficulties the victim must endure; education, inservice and interpretation of the pathophysiological sequelae; and ramifications for future rehabilitation and therapy services, are also offered.

Depending on the need, we can provide a brief, moderate, or comprehensive medical review. We can review cases for merit, provide a chronology and summary of the complete medical record, hospital policy and procedure, client interviews, disease process, reported diagnosis, prognosis, delivered healthcare, and standards of practice. This review includes recommendations and conclusions which are fully documented. Copies of all referral sources are included with the report.

We provide the attorney with a comprehensive, cost-and time-efficient service. All cases are reviewed by professional, experienced legal nurses consultants who are experts in a variety of specialties. This enhances their effectiveness because they can identify specific deviations of care using current standards, practices, and procedures.

Someone once wrote that no matter what you do, no matter where you go, the secret to success is in developing your skill, knowing your client base, and keeping your overhead down.

Working at home and already possessing a complete computer system kept my overhead low. I had no additional rent or utilities except for an additional phone line, answering service, long distance calls, a fax machine, advertising costs, and associated expenses attending seminars and luncheons for networking with special interest groups (SIGS), attorney and CPA fees, and computer maintenance and subscription fees to national database information services like Compuserve, Medline, GEnie, Westlaw, etc.

You must find what is unique about yourself or your services that warrants selecting your company over someone else. If you do not know, then why should anyone use you? Check out your competition. Find out who they are, where they are, what they offer, and what they are charging. Base your fees below theirs, offer something extra for a discount, and let your clients know this. Let them know that you appreciate their business.

Listen carefully, be accessible at all times, and never give excuses. Do not complain to your client about being overworked, back-logged, or behind schedule. It is not their problem, and it tells them you are unable to perform your job, and they will remember that! Remember, repeat business is what you are going after, and they will be your source for the future referrals.

Write a business plan. Identify what you want to do, how you are going to do it, and why. This will help you develop your scope of practice and identify your prospective client base. Be sure to include what you will charge them, as well as how you are going to collect your fees. For new clients I have found it beneficial to get at least 75 percent payment up front. This will keep your cash flow up and will help to weed out deadbeats. Do not forget to list what your qualifications are to perform your services. This will help you and your banker, attorney and CPA determine your marketability and your potential for success.

Make use of all available resources from your profession organizations: clubs, local libraries, college or universities, and your peers. Network with others for different ideas and use their contracts. Always use a referral name when contacting new or prospective clients. It will help you get your foot in the door.

Stay in touch with your clients. Attend functions that are geared toward developing your client base. Mingle with them and pass out plenty of your cards. Do not rely on "cold calling."

When designing your home office make sure that it is in an area that is comfortable for you to work in and can be used exclusively for work. Your office needs to be spacious enough so that you can work relatively clutter-free, have adequate lighting, be free of distraction, and be easy to keep clean and tidy.

Experiment with the design of your office furniture and equipment. My office layout is in a U-shape. This integrates an open, uncrowded accessibility with utility. Everything important is readily available. I do not feel crowded or closed in, so I can relax and focus on my work.

Chose your CPA and a small business attorney by their experience, success, and personality—not by their cost. The reason for this is that you must feel comfortable with whom you entrust your business' life blood, and you will save money in the long run by not having to pay for costly mistakes or for services that would take an inexperienced individual longer to do.

Keep detailed records of all expenses. Get to know the IRS and CPA intimately. Make sure that you can justify all expenses claimed on your returns. The IRS offers free small business workshops and assistance for home businesses. Take advantage of them by contacting your local IRS office or call their toll free number at 800-424-1040. The key to successful tax savings and deductions is at the time you make your purchase, not at the end of the tax year.

If you decide to enter, or are already in, the business of medical-legal consulting, there are some important points to remember. Be careful how you approach the development of your business. I was working as an agency nurse while I was developing my business, and I did not want to be labeled as a whistleblower or a hired gun. Hospital administrators and supervisors become paranoid and malicious when they hear that you do malpractice case review. Some facilities will try to ban you, as one did to me.

I was very upset and concerned when that happened. I was still in the designing stages of my business when one of the area hospitals found out. In the back of my mind I had heard of people doing this, but what would I do if I could not get any work anywhere else as a result of this? My wife just had our baby boy and had also recovered from a lengthy illness. I had responsibilities to them and bills to pay. I was definitely out on a limb, but the limb is the only place where the *fruit* is.

George Douglass once said that business failure from under-capitalization is a myth. The reality is that it is the result of improper tools, mismanagement, poor planning, or lack of commitment. Money is never a substitute for creativity, clever strategy, or doing what needs to be done when it needs to be done. I believe this emphatically. You must have the proper attitude, for attitude is the key to success.

MedLaw, Inc.
P.O. Box 744235
Dallas, TX 75374-4235
(214) 387-7848

Chapter 21

Improved Patient Outcome
and
Cost-Containment

(This profile appeared in the September 1990 issue of the *Nurse-Entrepreneur's Exchange*.)

Editor's Note : Material Resource Associates, Inc. (MRA), of Long Beach, California, was founded in 1987 by Vickie R. Fullerton, RN, BSN, along with her husband and partner, Stephen Fullerton. MRA provides healthcare cost-containment services and products to a variety of clients.

Fullerton's background, prior to starting MRA, includes working as a critical care clinician, manager, and educator.

NNE: What was your motivation for starting MRA?
Vickie: "Back in 1985, I began to seriously wonder if there was life after acute care. I felt a defiance for the acute-care system, and decided if I didn't make a change, I would be leaving nursing altogether. As many nurses do, I felt caught between a rock and a hard place, with nowhere else to go.

One of the biggest problems I had with hospital nursing is that I feel very creative and like to take a lot of risks. I wanted to make decisions and see the outcome of those decisions. But with hospital nursing, you're quite limited—you either get fired, or at least are not appreciated for the work that you do. Historically, in the nursing profession, we have not really been decision makers. So the career path that I chose was to completely distance myself from hospital nursing."

NEE: What did you do?
Vickie: " An area I thought would be creative was cost-containment because when I was a manager, I became involved with DRG's quality assurance, and utilization review—but I never really got to see the outcomes. The only people who truly have an incentive to see outcomes in patient care are the ones writing the checks and paying the bills.

So, I went to work for a large cost-containment company and learned the trade. Two years later, they decided to subcontract out their hospital bill audit program because it was no longer profitable for such a large company to focus on such a small program. I wrote a proposal to take over that program, and subsequently was able to successfully negotiate a good contract. That gave MRA its first client."

NEE: What other services does MRA provide?
Vickie: "Besides the hospital bill audit program, offered to both private health insurance carriers and worker's compensation carriers, we also offer case management and utilization review."

NEE: What was your marketing approach?
Vickie: "I took a lot of training in marketing by attending seminars and classes, and learned the importance of developing a marketing plan to get my target market in focus. Our marketing plan included doing mass mailings to third-party administrators and self-insured companies. And it worked perfectly well.

What I did was to extend my product to a wider group of customers—and I did it quickly. Within three months of forming MRA, we developed our marketing plan, and initiated it in the form of the mailings and follow up."

NEE: Is there a difference in the approach of a case manager who works for an insurance company and an independent case management company such as MRA?
Vickie: "Yes. If you're a Blue Cross case manager, your loyalty is to Blue Cross to make sure you are not going to spend any more money than is necessary—sometimes to the point of sacrificing the actual delivery of patient care. An outside vendor can look at it more objectively, and provide the care necessary for a patient regardless of the cost, because we have no conflict of interest."

NEE: In that case, why would a carrier even use an outside vendor?
Vickie: "At this point in time, very few insurance companies do their own case management. They stay away from providing direct cost-containment products and services, primarily because there are some antitrust issues involved. They don't want to be accused of any conflict of interest from their client's perspective."

NEE: What makes MRA's services unique?
Vickie: "We focus on the needs of clients. Our services are very customized, and I believe in the philosophy of sharing risks with clients.

We're a completely fee-for-service company, with no hidden costs. We also stick with the turn-around time that we promise our clients. So we are very consistent with our time frame and our pricing. I also make it a point to personally visit every one of our clients. They may know you through letters and phone calls, but it's different when you meet them face to face. It creates a bonding—almost like a mother/child relationship.

We also provide a customized reporting system. If a client wants a specific report, we will take all the available information and design a report that is user-friendly. We have a standardized reporting system, but if a client needs something different, we will accommodate them."

NEE: Are you enjoying what you do with MRA?
Vickie: "I am! I'm very excited and hyper. I spend a lot of hours and work very hard, but I really enjoy what I do. I can't say I have tons of money, but I have clothes on my back, a roof over my head, and I don't owe anyone any money.

In this kind of business, we were able to get the business going and have it support itself. We did not have to get a loan, or utilize all our earnings to put into the business, because what we have is a service product. And with a service product, you spend time and energy, but the actual dollar cost is minimal."

NEE: Any tips for nurses starting a business?
Vickie: "Before you jump into anything, design a good business plan and know exactly what your marketing strategy is going to look like.

Also, utilize the resources available to you. If you don't know how to market, get someone who knows how to market. It may cost some money to get an initial consultation, but at least you'll be doing it the right way. This is one way that NNBA has been very good to all of us—we have the nurses who have experience who can teach the newer ones going into business.

The way that changes happen is to become actively involved. If you want to get into business, you can fantasize about it until the cows come home, but until you act, it's not going to happen.

I've never felt as good a nurse as I have since starting my business. I can actually quantify patient outcome."

UPDATE 1997

Victoria Rodriguez Fullerton co-founded MRA, Inc. in January, 1989 to offer Insurance Cost Containment services including hospital bill audit and medical peer review programs to self-insured employers. MRA now offers a full range of services in utilization management, medical case management, bill validation, post discharge review, disability management, benefit plan design and consultation to self-insureds, government agencies, and plan administrators. As the President of MRA, Ms. Fullerton is responsible for overseeing the marketing and development of the company's programs as well as MRA's quality assurance program.

In January, 1996, Ms. Fullerton was elected to a four year term on the Board of Directors of the Case Management Society of America (CMSA) and appointed to the Board of Directors of the Legal Aid Foundation of Long Beach. In May, 1996, Ms. Fullerton was appointed to the Board of Directors of the State Assistance Fund for Enterprise, Business and Industrial Development Corporation (SAFE-BIDCO). Ms. Fullerton is a Founding Sister of the Asian Pacific American Women's Leadership Institute.

She is an active board member of the National Association of Women Business Owners, Los Angeles (NAWBO-LA) and the California American Woman's Economic Development Corporation (AWED). Ms. Fullerton is also a member of the Democratic National Committee. In 1994, Ms. Fullerton was honored by AWED as their nominee for "Business Owner of the Year" at the National Association of Women in Business Owners (NAWBO) annual meeting. Ms. Fullerton serves as a member of the Private Industry Council of the City of Long Beach, sits on the Blue Ribbon Advisory Committee of Women incorporated, and she was a California delegate to the 1995 White House Conference on Small Business. Ms. Fullerton is a past board member of the Long Beach West End Community Association

Material Resource Associates, Inc.
110 Pine, Suite 525
Long Beach, CA 90802
(310) 437-4331

147

Chapter 22

Let's Get Down To Business: The Story of N.P.A.

by Margretta Kray, RNC, ANP, and Valerie Nielsen, RNC, ANP

There is no better impetus for starting your own business than finding yourself without a job.

After years of working in educational positions in a hospital setting and finding ourselves moving farther away from patient care, we determined to make a change that would bring us back to the patient. To accomplish this, we enrolled together in a nurse practitioner program, taking a leave of absence from our current positions. Our plan was to return to the hospital in a new capacity, equipped with advanced clinical skills.

Near the completion of our program, we returned to the hospital to discuss possible roles. These words still echo, "I'm sorry, you're better off on the inside in any capacity than you are on the outside." Due to budget cutbacks that had occurred during our year's leave of absence, the position "on the inside" was that of a nursing assistant! We chose "the outside" with no regrets.

With hours of commute time in a car on our way to and from school in another city, we began to brainstorm about options for employment. It was logical to approach a primary care facility about adding two nurse practitioners to their staff. Each attempted contact, though, was a dead end with comments like, "We"ll keep your applications on file." Our interpretation of these encounters was that existing providers viewed us as a threat. No one was willing to listen to the possibilities for an expanded nursing role. Picture this interview with a physician who refused to sit and talk, but instead had to stand and pace, muttering all the while about taking business away from physicians!

The realization that we really were "on the outside" became increasingly apparent. School was over; we were graduates with new skills, full of ideas and enthusiasm, and no jobs. We were on our own, and if we were to have employment, we'd have to find ways to make it happen ourselves.

On the front porch in the early morning hours, before our children were awake for the day, we began exploring possibilities for creating a nursing business. After much reading, research, and discussion, the way became clear: we formed a partnership called Nurse Practitioner Associates (N.P.A.)

There were few resources for starting a nursing business back in 1984. Dayani and Riccardi's book, *The Nurse Entrepreneur* (Reston Publishing Co., Reston, VA, 1982), was very helpful, along with our accountant. Finding an attorney who was well versed on nursing businesses was not easy. In fact, we're on our third one now, who happens to have been an RN, shows interest, and has the knowledge concerning healthcare professionals in business. Fortunately, the need for an attorney has been more of a formality than a necessity.

To keep our overhead low we decided to work out of our homes. We do all the secretarial work and have been able to continue this system because our services always take us to other sites which provide facilities for our use.

Selection of a name for our business was an important issue, since it reflects both our role and identity. We wanted it to be just right! Over the years, however, we've noticed that others don't consider our name quite as significant, as shown by the various mailing labels we have received. Here are some rather humbling examples:

Norse Practitioner Associates
Nurd Practitioner Associates
Nurse Practitioner Ass

N.P.A. is a business that contracts with other agencies to provide services such as: assessment and nursing management of adult health problems, health teaching, health counseling, professional education, consultation, and wellness programs. When we began, we provided services for a family planning clinic, and to fill in we provided insurance physicials and patient teaching for diabetics in a neighboring community clinic.

After a year or so, we changed our focus to wellness and designed a program for business and industry. We called the program "WELL-THY; Stay Well and Healthy," and registered it as our own trademark. The program offers individual health risk assessment, individual counseling sessions to work on behavior change, and group classes tailored to the group profile of the participating business. N.P.A. provides all activities at the worksite. The wellness program was perfect for us to develop, since it required no physician involvement, and has given access to a variety of non-traditional settings for nurses. A bonus was the opportunity to work with well clients.

Continuing education classes and workshops for nurses is another area we have been able to develop. We market our workshops via letters, personal contacts, and referrals for universities, hospitals, and technical colleges,who then co-sponsor the events. We've served several communities in Southern Minnesota and South Dakota and enjoy the opportunities for travel. Our favorite workshop topic is Therapeutic Touch, which provides a delightful experiential day for the participants and the presenters.

Our primary clinical role occurs through a contract with a regional treatment center that offers psychiatric, chemical dependency, and adolescent services. We provide admission, annual, discharge, and female health exams for the clientele. We continue to explore other avenues for expansion of services, such as employee health services and the parish nurse concept. There's always something brewing on the back burner since the opportunities are almost limitless!

A critical issue in starting our own business was to have a strong support system. We were fortunate to have interested and supportive families who understood our dreams and desires to venture out on our own. It was equally important that the two of us could share successes as well as the setbacks. We've been able to support each other. We strongly encourage anyone who is starting their own business to identify a support person at the outset. Networking helps provide needed support and becomes an invaluable marketing tool. We attended the first annual National Nurses in Business Association conference and found out that, indeed, there are others out there.

Marketing is a new concept for most nurses in business. View every article, every personal contact as a potential opportunity for expanding services. Newspapers are full of stories about needs that exist within society. Who can meet those needs? Which needs warrant new services? Be creative as you consider how your own business can build and grow along with our society.

Newspaper articles and television news stories are free publicity for your business. Write letters to the editor of your newspaper or TV station to interest them in finding out about your innovative business. It might cause stage fright, but it offers wide exposure at no cost.

One of the best ways to help yourself is to help someone else. Other hopeful nurse entrepreneurs are out there and could use a word of encouragement. One of the ways we've found to help other nurses is by a workshop we provide that focuses on ow to start a business.

Has N.P.A been a success? Yes! Would we do it again? Yes! Are we glad we chose to be on "the Outside?" Yes! Actually, we're not on the outside anymore; we're on the inside of a progressive nursing business.

UPDATE 1997

Nurse Practitioner Associates has continued to thrive, and in 1994 celebrated its tenth anniversary! When we began NFA, we pledged to "give it a try," never dreaming we would be able to last ten years, and even longer!

Clinical services continue as the primary focus of our business. We now provide five-day coverage at the regional treatment center previously mentioned, and have expanded to cover a juvenile detention center. At that site we provide admission physical examinations, along with sick call. We look forward to further expansion of our clinical role with the addition of prescriptive privileges later this year.

There are always new opportunities for development of the business. One of these is the parish nurse role, which has been on the "back burner" for years. We're both preparing ourselves to function in that new role, as it evolves within our community.

About one day per month we schedule a continuing education event. Over the years our marketing techniques for these have changed considerably. Rather than sending letters and follow-up calls, we now receive numerous requests, and have the luxury of selecting those opportunities we prefer. It seems our reputation is established as a quality and reliable provider, therefore, we need to spend much less time in marketing activities.

Over the years we've appreciated the peer support of each other within the partnership, of other nurse practitioners, and advanced practice nurses. We are pleased to note these groups have increased in numbers and visibility in our locale. The caring support of our families continues to be an important factor in the success of NPA.

We look forward to another decade of successful nurse entrepreneurship with NPA!

Nurse Practitioner Associates
725 S.W Sixth Street
Willmar, MN 56201
(612) 235-7790

Chapter 23

Optimal Employee Health Through Screening

(This profile appeared in the July 1989 issue of the *Nurse-Entrepreneur's Exchange.*)

Editor's Note: After graduating from nursing school in 1979, James Slover, RN, BSN, began working as an ER nurse. Less than a year later, in 1980, he founded HealthCheck, Inc., in Topeka, Kansas. HealthCheck, Inc. provides health screening services to insurance companies, government agencies, employers, and the military.

NEE: Why did an ER nurse decide to establish a health screening company?
Jim: "I made a decision that I didn't want to work in the hospital—I have an aversion to punching somebody else's timeclock. Plus, when I found myself working on Christmas Day for straight pay, I decided it wasn't for me. I needed to do something else, but didn't have much of a clinical background to base any kind of nursing business on since I was a new grad. So, I started looking around to find something I could do with my nursing credential that did not require an extensive clinical background. Health screening for insurance companies was an area I felt I could get into."

NEE: What was your first step?
Jim: "I checked out the marketplace to see what was going on. There were two companies in town providing services, one of which was

doing a good job, but wasn't aggressive in their marketing. The other folks were aggressive marketers, but did a poor job of delivering services. That company started going down the tubes due to poor management—I came in just as they were starting to fail, so I filled the niche."

NEE: Good timing!
Jim: "Yes. Hard work is a requirement of course, but luck has a lot to do with business, no matter what anyone tells you. Also, while I was in nursing school, I worked for a man who was an entrepreneur. I got the chance to see how to run a business for yourself, and what it takes to make it go. Truthfully, if I had not had that experience I probably would not have been successful.

I opened up for business on January 2, 1980. We did very little business for the first two months, but I kept busy doing a lot of one-on-one marketing. Again, this other firm that I was in competition with was doing such a poor job that the people I was calling on were very ready to make a change. So, business gradually picked up, but it took a year and a half before I was able to pay myself a salary."

NEE: Did the startup phase progress smoothly?
Jim: "Oh no. I made some mistakes early on—I tried to grow too quickly. When you're new in business, you tend to go out and plant a bunch of seeds and see what grows. I had several colleagues who wanted to do something in nursing, so we attempted to start a home health agency. It failed due to lack of funding. I also had an exceptionally talented nurse that worked for me—he went out and marketed and installed an occupational health nursing program. So we were trying to get a fledgling home care agency off the ground and doing occupational health nursing for a major firm here in Topeka.

Basically, I got overextended and just couldn't do it all. So I made the decision that we were going to do what we do best, and what would generate the most output for the input, i.e,: how we were going to make the most money for the amount of time spent—and that was health screening services."

NEE: What specific services does HealthCheck, Inc. provide?
Jim: "We provide health screening services largely to insurance companies, which consists of a detailed health history, vital signs, height/weight and urine tests. Depending on the amount of insurance, they might require blood tests which typically include a chem profile, an AIDS test and a drug screen. We also do EKG's, CXR's, and pulmonary function studies.

If you get into substantial amounts of insurance, or you have a health history, they may want to have a physician take a look at you. I have physicians that function as independent contractors working for me to perform complete history and physicals.

We also provide screening services to state and federal agencies. We do virtually all the intake physicals for the state's vocational rehab program here in Topeka. In addition, we provide screening services to the military, which has turned out to be a very lucrative end of the business."

NEE: HealthCheck provides the military induction physicals?
Jim: "No. Everyone in the National Guard is required to have a physical exam every four years. They had been using traditional sources in the medical community to get those done, but the medical community is not willing to toe the line when it comes to government paperwork—you have to do it right the first time, or you're back to square one. We pay attention to getting the paperwork completed properly and have a rapid turn-around time.

We also put a heavy emphasis on convenience, especially for the military physicals. These people work on the weekend, so we pack up a road show, go to them and set up a mini-clinic onsite where they are drilling, and perform the physicals on government time."

NEE: Where do you find the MD's who contract with HealthCheck?
Jim: "The Menninger Foundation here in Topeka is one of the premier psychiatric learning institutions in the world, and I've been able to tap into the resident physician population there. These are folks who make a subsistence salary—they can come into my office and make $40-$80 an hour doing physicals and get paid on the spot. They like that real well. My attitude is that I want to pay people well, so they want to come and want to work. This way I don't have to run around looking for new people all the time.

We also provide screening services for local employers, primarily pre-employment physicals. That's an area of the business that I am going to be developing more extensively—we haven't done much marketing in this area, but there is certainly much room for growth."

NEE: Speaking of growth, how has HealthCheck grown?
Jim: "Our firm has experienced a 20-40 percent growth rate every year for the past six or seven years. We did about $100,000 last year, and we're running 10-15 percent more than that so far this year.

A large part of what we sell is physician services. That's not to say that nurses can't do good physicals, but they are not acceptable to the government. Also, the medical directors of insurance companies are doctors, and they are not about to accept a nurse's assessment.

We've also consulted with firms on occupational health issues, such as how to reduce worker's compensation costs. And the way to accomplish that is by having an occupational health nurse in-house. There is a tremendous opportunity for nurses to work for corporations in this area. It's a very labor intensive area and the docs don't want it. Not only is the nurse in there to treat on-the-job injuries, but they also prevent injuries by conducting health education programs.

Looking at the healthcare system in a macro sense, corporations have been trying to control healthcare costs with mechanisms such as HMO's and PPO's. That is just cost shifting—it doesn't reduce the size of the pie, it just decides who is going to get what piece. What we, as nurses, are able to do is reduce the size of that pie. We can reduce demand by helping people to be healthier, and that's a long-term project.

The best way to do that is to have a nurse in the workplace—you have to go to the people. You have to be a ready resource for information and assessment. Corporations have the motivation to provide that kind of service because they're paying the health insurance bill. Some people say. 'I don't want to go to some nurse when I can go to my doc—he's got a medical degree and all this experience.' But once people experience what nurses are capable of doing, they understand that what they're getting is a higher level of healthcare—not less, but more."

NEE: What current marketplace challenges does HealthCheck face?
Jim: "There is an unfortunate reality with paramedical service companies like myself, which is that the major insurance companies are shrinking the number of firms that they've approved to do business with. What's happening is this—there are about a dozen major national paramedical firms. These firms have got examiners in every nook and cranny around. So, the insurance companies can negotiate rates on a national basis—they got one bill instead of a hundred—and if they have quality control problems, they have only one person they need to call. Logistically, I understand why they do it. On the other hand, if the insurance companies' clients had the same attitude when they were starting out, they wouldn't be in business today.

To circumvent that, what we have done is to continue to do as much business as possible as HealthCheck, then, for the past five years we have been brokering business through one of the national paramedical companies. I have to cut them a third of my fees just for the use of their name, but it does allow me to be of service to anybody. It has

159

been less than 10 percent of our gross volume that we've had to broker through these companies, so it hasn't made that big of a dent in our business."

NEE: Any advice you can offer the beginning nurse in business?
Jim: "Don't try to do it all yourself. Don't try to understand all the government regulations and do all your own bookkeeping. I don't like paying an accountant $50 an hour, but I'd rather do that than lose sleep and pay penalties because things weren't filed properly. Make good use of attorneys and accountants and get your business established properly from day one. It's real hard to backtrack and correct your problems—it is money well spent to hire those professionals."

UPDATE 1997

Our business continues to operate much as it has since 1980. We are doing an increasing volume of employment related drug testing. Health screening services can be an excellent stand alone operation or an adjunct to other nursing services. I am available as a consultant to those interested in setting up this type of business.

HealthCheck, Inc.
1525 S. Topeka, Suite A
Topeka, KS 66612
(913)233-5535

Chapter 24

Professional Speaking for Fun and Profit

by Patty Wooten, BSN, CCRN

After fifteen years as a critical care nurse, I decided I wanted to have more fun on the job, or at least to recognize the fun and funny aspects. I had been a practicing clown for many years and wanted to explore the effects of clowning on the elderly residents in a nursing home.

The activities director was quite pleased at my offer to volunteer my time and talents, and in exchange for my efforts, she agreed to observe and record the changes in the residents' behavior or mood. We found residents had an increased response and interaction with the clown and between each other after the clown's visit. This stimulated my curiosity, and I began a library search for others who had explored the powerful effects of humor and laughter. Norman Cousins had written *Anatomy of an Illness*, showing how effective laughter was for his recovery from ankylosing spondylitis. I felt encouraged by the discovery of an important link between laughter and recovery from illness. Because I had the skills of a professional nurse and the talents of an entertaining clown, I continued to visit nursing homes and hospitals in my community.

Over the years, I've learned to stay open to the suggestions and advice of people I respect and trust. My director of nursing at the time suggested I contact her friend, who was the chairman of the nursing department at the local community college.

The chairman described how he'd instituted a "Caring Curriculum" to begin instructing nursing students about the art of caring. He requested that I speak to them about how humor could be a self-care tool to help nurses cope with job stress and burnout. I felt challenged by his request to create an educational format for what had, up to that time, been interactive and spontaneous. The students enjoyed the presentation, but I knew I could make it even better with more information, so I attended the very first "Laughter and Play" conference by the Institute for the Advancement of Human Behavior.

The opening keynote was by Norman Cousins, and we met briefly, but my big opportunity came when I met a woman who owned her own nursing education business. Nurses had been requesting that she write a workshop on the healing power of humor. She offered me the chance to do that and then teach it for her. It was the perfect way for me to start. Her confidence in my abilities inspired me to risk trying something I'd never done before. Her business could do the advertising, scheduling, and fee collection—I would be free to create.

Along with many hours of library research and telephone networking with other humor consultants, I created "Nancy Nurse," a nurse-clown character, to portray the outrageously funny events that occur in nursing. At first, I would only teach two or three days each month, so I continued working at the hospital part-time. I began teaching around California, and as the popularity for the workshop grew, I began working per diem when my income required a boost.

After two years I decided to go out on my own. Up to that time, I'd taught primarily in California, with a great response. I suspected that the market could be national. I developed my own brochure with advice from some friends in marketing, read the book *Guerrilla Marketing*, and wrote to every state nursing association, state hospi-

162

tal association, and national professional nursing association, submitting a brochure and cover letter. I began receiving calls and booking presentations.

As the audiences grew larger, I realized that I needed more skills and polish to make my presentation more professional, so I joined the National Speakers Association and began learning techniques for making a powerful impact on audiences, as well as tips on marketing, record keeping, and networking.

They suggested that you promote your business at every opportunity, even when the immediate benefit doesn't seem obvious. I began giving my business cards to friends, asking that they share them with whoever they thought might be interested. I gave one to a friend who was vacationing in Maine, who passed it along to her friend whose brother was working in rural health education.

About a month later, I received a call from the program director at Medical Care Development. He was delighted to hear of my work and was planning a video conference on "Humor and Health" to be aired into hospitals across the nation via the satellite system. He'd already booked Norman Cousins and was looking for health professionals to create a panel; would I be interested? This was the second big break for my business.

Because of my networking, I had become acquainted with physicians, nurses, and researchers who'd been exploring the effects of humor. I gathered a panel of experts, and we all went off to Hollywood for filming, which was broadcast in 800 facilities in thirty-six states. Two weeks after that, I mailed my brochure and cover letter to each facility that had viewed the video conference.

Today, only six years after that first nursing school presentation, I am speaking nationally about six to eight times each month. My workshop "Jest for the Health of It" has been presented in forty-two states and Canada. I've been filmed for British television, and in the summer of 1990, I traveled to England to present the results of my research at the Eighth International Conference on Humor. My research studied the effect of humor training for nurses to modify their symptoms of burnout.

I also write a regular column for the *Journal of Nursing Jocularity*, a new quarterly journal of nursing humor. I am preparing to expand my services to include clown training classes and consulting on establishing humor rooms or comedy carts in hospitals.

If I were asked for advice about beginning a speaking/consulting business, I'd say pick a focus that is unique and something you really enjoy, have experience in, and are curious about exploring. So often the motivation to continue through difficult times has to come from within, and if you're not excited or having fun, it's hard to convey the importance of your message to others. Next, I'd suggest finding a mentor—someone who is already doing similar work to what you are considering.

Continue your development through seminars, reading, and professional associations. Realize that your profession has now expanded beyond the bedside activities, so your development may include marketing strategies, record keeping, or speaking skills.

Always appear professional. If your office is in your home, have a separate line from the family's, and always be available through an answering machine or service. I find the remote call retrieval option very important if you arc traveling out of town for several days. Be sure that any paperwork that represents your business has professional polish. Phone and written correspondence are often the only clues your client has about the quality of your work.

That old adage, *dress for success*, is important. A professional speaker once advised me to remember: "When a man stands up to speak, they listen to what he has to say and may notice what he is wearing, but when a woman stands up to speak, they notice what she's wearing and then decides whether they want to listen." This reveals the sexist nature of our society, but if you want to win the game, you've got to remember the rules.

Next, realize that you can't do everything yourself (a difficult concept for all of us "super nurses" to grasp), and hire a part-time assistant to keep meticulous records of all your contacts and financial activity. Once this gets out of control, it's a major pain to try to recover it. Early on, I suffered from computer phobia. Now, I truly appreciate how efficient it makes my record keeping. Also, I suggest getting a professional tax preparation person who is familiar with tax laws. My final advice is to forgive yourself when you make mistakes, learn from them, and then move on, revising your actions to avoid them in the future.

I've learned many lessons during these last six years, and probably the greatest of these is that my service is worth a lot more than I ever suspected. People are willing to pay for quality, so I keep myself informed about what fees other national speakers are commanding. Never publish your fee schedule; always discuss this on the phone after you have assessed their needs, size of audience, and type of facility. I always try to be flexible with my fees and help them solve funding problems by suggesting other resources, such as vendor sponsors, auxiliary assistance, co-sponsoring the program with a nearby facility, or adding an evening talk for the community to bring attention to the hospital.

When invited to speak at a national convention, realize that this is an incredible marketing opportunity that will generate other engagements. I will drastically lower my fees for the exposure I will receive, though I request that the office refer all inquiries about my work directly to me. I have also learned to request a referral letter about the response to my workshop, as well as copies of participant evaluations and comments. I can use these in the future if people request references. The best overall advertisement is word-of-mouth from participants, therefore I always have my address and phone number on several places in the handout, as well as having brochures and business cards available.

My quest six years ago was to find more fun in my work and to discover the funny aspects of nursing. I didn't plan to be a nationally recognized expert on humor and health, but as my path unfolded before me, I tried to recognize and potentiate each opportunity.

Sometimes I would "fake it until I made it," accepting an assignment, and then diligently preparing myself for the challenge and adapting along the way—but then I've been doing that as a bedside nurse for more than twenty years, so it was already part of my nature.

UPDATE 1997

Wow, has it been six years already since I wrote the first version of my adventure as a nurse entrepreneur? Whew, so much has happened in such a short time. I was delighted when Laura Gasparis Vonfrolio asked me to update my chapter to include the new information and lessons I learned since 1991.

In the last six years, I've written and published two books, produced three video programs, started a product line of humor supplies, served as president of the American Association for Therapeutic Humor, appeared on many TV and radio shows, and have been featured in a half page article with photos in USA Today (October 31, 1996). This level of success has been reached because of commitment, networking and just plain hard work. I firmly believe that if you truly believe in the importance of your message or service, you will find the energy, enthusiasm and creativity that every entrepreneur needs to succeed.

And yet, if I had learned some important lessons earlier in my career, I would be even more successful. I now share some of these lessons with you in the hope that it will catapult your business to greater success. The areas I will discuss are networking, marketing and product development.

The Power of Networking

My daddy once told me, as I trekked off to college, "It's not what you know, it's who you know." I resented that statement as I eagerly began my quest for knowledge, but now, almost 30 years later, I have discovered that "who you know" can be extremely helpful.

I suggest that you begin to gather business cards, brochures, e-mail addresses, fax numbers of any and everyone you meet as you develop your business. Next find computer database programs to manage this information. One of the best I've found is A.C.T. (available in both PC and Macintosh) and costs about $100. This program will help you control all aspects of information related to your clients and contacts. You can arrange them into specialty groups, search for names by different criteria, fax directly from the program, create a dated list of calls, tasks and meetings you need to do and then sent set an alarm to remind you to do them. When you create a letter, proposal, fax or anything else, you can attach it to the contact file so that when you pull up that contact, you have a copy and dated list of every call and correspondence you've had with that person. This kind of detailed organization is essential because as your business grows you will have a tremendous amount of information to keep track of and you always need to be accurate and organized with your clients.

Now that you're organized, remember to stay in touch with your contacts via postcards, newsletters and e-mail. I cannot emphasize enough the importance of getting "online" if at all possible. If you have a computer and a modem, you can obtain an internet account for as little as $20 per month. This will allow you to maintain contact with anyone, in any place in the world for just pennies per day. Business today moves rapidly and information is often required quickly; an internet connection will allow you to quickly and easily communicate with people. You can also use the internet to provide added value and service to your customers or to advertise your business. I have an e-mail list of people I call my "Humor Pals." I can easily send out funny stories or papers with just a few keystrokes. It takes only moments and costs nothing. This low cost "added value service" is a gentle reminder to my friends and customers of who I am and the purpose and value of my message about Humor and Well-being.

Networking depends on being organized, staying connected and sharing ideas with colleagues. I also suggest that you join one or more professional organizations related to your business topics. I'm a member of the American Association for Therapeutic Humor and the International Society for Humor Studies. These affiliations keep me up to date with new developments in my field and provide opportunities to share ideas and projects with experts. Offer to speak at conventions and write articles for journals related to your business specialty. This will help to establish you as an expert in your field and may lead to media exposure which will help to promote your business, which leads me to the next "lesson" I want to share.

The Power of Marketing

The truth about success is...no matter how good you are, if no one knows about you, your business won't grow. Six years ago when I wrote this chapter, I talked of the power of "word of mouth" advertising. While that is possibly the best kind, I don't recommend that you depend on it. I did, and it was a BIG mistake. Sure, my business did grow, but not nearly as large or rapidly as it could have if I'd had a marketing plan or marketing skills.

I've recently learned about the power of "benefit driven copy." This is an advertising term which means: describe your business first in terms of the customer benefits and then in terms of the service you provide and why you are qualified. This technique will immediately "hook" the customers and pull them into the story about your business because they know the BENEFITS you can provide for them. Another advertising concept to consider is called USP or Unique Selling Position. Ask yourself, how is your service different from your competitors, why are you unique among others providing a similar service or product. And finally, be sure you have "targeted" your market. Analyze who can utilize your service based on your USP and then begin your marketing attempts with that group.

For example, my USP is that I am a nurse with clinical experience in a wide variety of different specialties. I am also a clown and skilled humorist. Therefore, my beginning "target market" was nursing organizations and hospital staff development departments. Since then, I have branched into patient support groups, human service professionals and community groups interested in humor and health. My "benefit driven copy" has phrases such as "Productivity and communication improve when employees have fun while they work." "Patients report greater satisfaction when care is delivered with a smile and a positive attitude." "Scientific research proves that laughter strengthens the immune system." Remember, your USP, targeted market and benefit driven copy will increase the effectiveness of any marketing you do.

The Power of Product Development

Whether you are a service business or an information business (like me) you can enhance your service and your income by providing products that are related to your business. For my business, these products include books, audio tapes, video tapes, funny props and Mirth Aid Kits. Sometimes the cost of these products is included in with the service I provide and other times they are sold separately. They can be sold by mail order as well as at the time of service (back of room sales). These products can also be bundled together and offered at a discounted rate. You can offer these products as a prize from a drawing of business cards, which you will then add to your data base to promote future services or a product catalogue.

The obvious benefit of product sales is increased income, but a hidden benefit is an increased perception of you as an expert and a "full service" business. Be sure to obtain a resale license from your State Board of Equalization and collect the appropriate sales tax from your state. I also suggest that you maintain your financial records in a computer program such as Quicken. If you create a catalogue (no matter how small) you can also promote your products while you market for your service.

Well, those are the big pearls of wisdom I've gained in the last six years as a nurse entrepreneur. I hope that you will find them helpful and effective. If you need more information, books by Jeffrey Lant are an excellent source. Remember, the keys to your success are energy, enthusiasm and creativity. Focus your efforts on networking, marketing and product development. Good luck and let me know how you're doing.

Jest for the Health of It
P.O. Box 4040
Davis, CA 95617
(916) 758-3826
fax: (916) 753-7638
e-mail: jestpatty@mother.com

Chapter 25

Promoting Political Action

(This profile appeared in July 1990 issue of the *Nurse-Entrepreneur's Exchange.*)

Editor's Note: Sharp Legislative Resources is a Washington, D.C. based company established in 1990 to assist nurses to their education on healthcare legislation and regulation, global health policy, and the federal legislative and regulatory processes.

Founded by Nancy J. Sharp, RN, MSN, last January, programs available included a six-day Internship in Washington, D.C., a 1-3 day Health Policy Workshop, and a Leadership Development program, designed for elected officers and professional staff of nursing associations.

Sharp's background includes service as a co-founder, editor of the **Legislative Network for Nurses**, *a bimonthly newsletter, Director of Practice and Legislation for NAACOG, and Program Director for the National Federation for Specialty Nursing Organizations (NFSNO).*

NEE: Why did you establish Sharp Legislative Resources?
Nancy: "Until last year, I was program director of the Nurse in Washington Internship Program for the NFSNO. The Federation Internship Program committee, composed of six members from six specialty organizations, all had paid staff people working on the six-year program.

They decided to contract the program out, in order to become more cost-effective. So they sent out a Request for Proposals. I bid on it, and they gave me the contract in January."

NEE: Describe the six-day Internship Program.
Nancy: "We take a group, up to a maximum of 100 nurses, and each day has a focus. Sunday is Orientation Day, where everyone introduces themselves and tells why they came to Washington. We also go through the program syllabus.

Monday is Health Policy Day. We have speakers address the issue of why nurses, women, and all people, should be involved in the health policy-setting process.

Tuesday is Coalition Day. We have speakers that talk about why small associations need to develop into coalitions with other groups such as consumers, doctors, the public, and other nursing organizations. We also go to the White House for a briefing, where two or three administration officials talk to us about the healthcare issues of the day. That evening we have a special dinner called Nurse in Washington Roundtable. That's a dinner group that meets all the time, so, during the Internship Program we have the usual Washington group of around 100, plus the 100 nurse interns. We have a Congress person who comes and speaks at that dinner.

Wednesday is Capitol Hill Day. Before they get here, all of the 100 nurses will have made appointments to see their two Senators and Representatives. Everyone enjoys Wednesday—they love to be on Capitol Hill. They also go to hearings and get to see Committee Chairman, etc.

Thursday is Federal Agency Day. We have speakers talk about how Federal Agencies fit into this big process, and why nurses need to know about regulations and the rule-making process. In the afternoon we have small groups going out to various agencies. For example, the emergency department nurses are interested in seeing the Department of Transportation, since it is in charge of motorcycle helmet laws, etc. Nurse mid-wives might go to Health Care Finance Administration because they have reimbursement concerns.

Friday is State Day. In the morning speakers talk about successful legislative accomplishments in the states. After lunch the interns have a chance to write what we call a Political Action Plan, which outlines what they've learned over the past six days—then we adjourn.

Now, before they get here, they complete a Pre-Internship Survey, which asks what they've done in the way of political and legislative activity. Six months after they've been here, they get a survey that asks what they have done since, and what they've learned.

So it's a real learning experience, and people are very stimulated to continue in the legislative process and get more active. We tell them, 'Okay, this is how we do it, now you go home and get active in your state building coalitions and working for good legislation for yourselves, your community, and all the patients that you work with."

NEE: What is the cost of the Intern Program?
Nancy: "The fee is $600, plus the airfare and hotel. You can do the entire program for about $1,200."

NEE: How do you market the program?
Nancy: "We talk about it in specialty nursing organization newsletters and journals, and send out press releases."

NEE: Tell us about your 1-3 day Health Policy workshops.
Nancy: "Over the years, 750 people have come to the Intern Program. Of those, one group from Arizona got very enthusiastic, so they went home and created a Nurse in Arizona Roundtable. They also had in place something called the Arizona Nursing Network.

That was a coalition that included the Arizona SNA, rehab nurses, NACOOG nurses, and nurse anesthetists.

This group asked me to do a 'mini-internship' Washington program for approximately twenty nurses. Monday there will be speakers all day, and Tuesday we'll have breakfast with the entire Arizona congressional delegation. Wednesday will just be tourist stuff, and then they go home. So they get a mini-internship in two and a half days. Now that I have the model, I'll be offering this program to all the other states by sending a brochure to SNA's and nursing specialty organizations.

Additionally, I've been asked to write a monthly legislative column for the *Journal of Nursing Management*. I also do keynote speeches nationwide on the theme of how to get involved on a grassroots level."

NEE: What is the top national legislative issue that impacts on independent nursing practice?
Nancy: "Direct reimbursement for nursing services. We're making progress—nurse practitioners can now get paid through Medicaid. Geriatric nurse practitioners can get paid through Medicare, and nurse midwives can get paid under Medicare for doing gynecological exams. Now, all of this is influx because of the work that people are doing to get national health insurance, where all providers would be under the government system."

NEE: Do you think we'll be going to a national health insurance plan?
Nancy: "I think it's going to be a mix of public and private for America."

Sharp Legislative Resources
8819 Ridge Road
Bethesda, MD 20817
(301) 469-7150

Chapter 26

Recovery/Discovery: Conception To Now!

by Ann Marie Wyrsch, MS, RN, CS

I changed both my personal and my professional lifestyle within months of each other. I had been a Catholic nun for thirty-two years when I left the convent and married.

I had worked in institutions for about thirty-four years and knew I did not want to do that any longer. Changing my lifestyle was, without a doubt, the catalyst I needed to take the risk involved in leaving the institution and going into private practice. When I was no longer welcome where I had worked, I looked for creative options to earn a living.

I knew what I wanted to do. The target population I wanted to focus on was adult children of alcoholics. I wanted to help other adults recover from a limiting childhood and discover the power to live life more fully. I wanted to raise awareness of the depth and pervasiveness of growing up in a family with the disease of alcoholism (or some other dysfunction), and plant the seeds of empowerment that could blossom into a profound and comprehensive recovery.

What I did not know was how I could go about accomplishing this. I was aware that I had the assets I needed to build on. These assets included my personal and professional experience.

175

Personally, I had been actively recovering from growing up in a family with the disease of alcoholism. I am a recovering co-dependent.

Professionally, I had credentials that would be helpful. I had earned ANA certification as a clinical specialist in Psychiatric and Mental Health Nursing. I had extensive clinical experience and had attended many workshops.

I was able to build on these assets. The idea of how it could happen was conceived during a conversation with a nurse friend and colleague who had been counseling individual clients for a couple of years. She saw a need for them to learn new skills, particularly in a group setting. Of course, most of these persons had come from a family with alcoholism or some other dysfunction. What I had to offer was what she needed. She later provided me with a ready-made pilot group. She continues to refer many participants.

The idea of a structured educational-experiential series in a group setting was conceived. Slowly, the idea began to take form and evolve. I drew on wisdom and experience from many sources.

One of these experiences was having actively participated in many self-esteem seminars conducted by Jack Canfield. I now realize how he became a mentor for me. I had watched how his skills and confidence developed over a couple of years. At his first seminar which I attended, participants received a blank spiral notebook. At later seminars, participants received a three ring notebook with a logo and multiple handouts. I decided that he started "where he was," and continued to refine and improve his program. This was new to me.

Another valuable resource was my work with Rev. Peter Cambell, PhD and Rev. Edwin McMahon, PhD, of the Institute for Bio Spiritual Research. They offer workshops on "Bio-Spirituality Through Focusing," as originally developed by Eugene Gendlin of the University of Chicago. What I learned from them helped me to create a focusing atmosphere, one that was respectful of the process in each person. I was able to use a gentle, caring approach with them, and to teach participants to use that type of approach with themselves.

Without this awareness, I would probably have spent years in the gestation phase, planning and perfecting my first series. Instead, I drafted a broad outline of a twenty-week series, and just did it.

This new entity, an evolving business and a specific program, needed a name. I pondered names that would convey something of what it was all about. I chose Recovery/Discovery Consultants for the name of the business, and Recovery/Discovery Series for the name of the twenty-week program.

The newly named program was birthed when I met for the first time with twelve persons, all provided by my nurse-colleague friend, who agreed to be my pilot project. I stayed about a week ahead of the first group and shook through most of it.

Birth was only the beginning. I soon developed five nursing diagnoses for Co-dependence, using the format for nursing diagnoses in a then newly published book on nursing diagnosis. These diagnoses covered the areas of wounding: physical, emotional, mental, spiritual and social. I discovered that the interventions I was using addressed each of these areas. By organizing what I was doing in this format, I became even more clear and concise.

Initially, I had only a few handouts of the processes we used in class. By the seventh series, I had started using a notebook with handouts. Later, I added a lesson plan for each session.

Four years have passed, and the Recovery/Discovery Series continues to grow and develop. Original participants have referred spouses, parents, children, friends, and colleagues. The most "ready" participants are those who have noticed a change they liked in a person close to them.

Just a couple of years later, it is already hard to remember some of the challenges that seemed monumental at the time they happened. One of these was money.

Money, and charging for my services, was an area where I started at square one, and still need to continue to grow. I asked the pilot for a "voluntary" donation of $5.00 per session, and only one participant regularly "volunteered." I did learn by the second series to charge more, and not on a voluntary basis. (Although I now have a set fee, I have continued to offer a limited number of scholarships to persons who truly need them.)

Asking for a specific fee triggered many reactions in the participants. I still remember how I was devastated by a very bright young women. She vigorously attacked me in front of the whole group because I did not do this just "out of love." She wanted me to provide the unconditional love and nurturing she had gotten from her mother. Since my Achilles heel was just that, I had to do some work with myself. However, I became much clearer and stronger because of it. It was painful at the time, but most of my catastrophic expectations did not occur.

For example, I thought the whole group would agree with her at best, and all walk out at worst. Neither of the two happened. Instead, we did not pretend the challenge was not there, but dealt with it openly. It turned out to be healing, not only for me, but for most of the participants. Before the end of the series, there was another crisis about money with this woman. I was able to stay clear about her need to pay, gently but firmly. She was one of those who finished the series!

Another challenge was a computer. About three months into the first series, I admitted how useful a computer with a word processor could be. I got one. I cannot begin to describe the frustration I experienced in the beginning. My reaction ranged from wanting to cry because I felt so helpless about how to use it, to rage and wanting to kick it because I could not get it to do what I wanted.

I read books, made mistakes, asked questions, and persevered. I am fortunate to have a brother who is a computer whiz. He taught me more in a day than I learned by myself in months. I was again aware of the value of a teacher. I am now amazed at what I can do using word processing and enjoy several other programs I have added to my computer repertoire.

I continue to discover ways to more accurately and simply do my bookkeeping. Word processing has made it much easier to update the handouts I use. And the neat part is that I have only begun to tap the potential of what I can learn to do with the computer.

While my husband uses a program to keep the records needed for taxes, we have still found it necessary to retain a Certified Public Accountant for filing taxes because of the continuing changes the IRS makes.

The number of participants in each group of Recovery/Discovery Series is limited to twelve. Most of the groups have consisted of fewer than twelve. Participants have ranged in age from twenty-one to seventy-seven. Twenty-nine groups have completed the series, with a total of over 250 participants.

No two series, although the basic structure and format remain the same, are exactly alike. Each group, because it is made up of unique persons, develops its own personality and taps more deeply into different facets of recovery. I continue to learn from each participant and also continue to learn and grow from many outside sources.

Being without support from nurse colleagues was one of the most difficult parts of being on my own. I have recently learned of a newly formed local group of nurse entrepreneurs.

I started my own business at the age of fifty-three, in the midst of drastic lifestyle changes, I suspect that many others also start their own business when the "status quo" is irreconcilably shaken up. I would not change the timing for me, as I needed every life experience I had until the time Recovery/Discovery Consultants came into being. Since its beginning, I have achieved tremendous satisfaction from the growth I have experienced and from the growth I have witnessed in participants.

A summary of some of the most important lessons I've learned would include:
The need to take action and then develop the service, rather than trying to solve all problems before they even occur; the value of persevering in looking for someone who knows more than I do in a particular area, rather than spending valuable time floundering; the need for the support, inspiration, and example of other enterprising nurses; and, more compelling: *it's never too late to have a dream and follow it.*

UPDATE 1997

Facilitating Recovery/Discovery and being a Nurse Entrepreneur was the most difficult, most rewarding, and most personally and professionally fulfilling time of my entire career as a nurse. I facilitated thirty-two twenty week Recovery/Discovery groups over a five year period, in addition to using Bio-Spiritual Focusing in my work with clients. I retired at the end of 1993 mainly because I changed my priorities. My husband was diagnosed with End Stage Renal Disease early in 1992. We have no family geographically close and I chose to be free to companion him in the frequent mini-crises he has had since.

Before retiring, because of my extensive experience with facilitating Recovery/Discovery groups and my Bio-Spiritual Focusing background, I was privileged to co-present a four hour videotaped series entitled

"Learning the Focusing Steps" with Peter Campbell, Ph.D of the Institute for Bio-Spiritual Research. I am still teaching through this series. It is used to train Bio-Spiritual Focusing Facilitators in many states. It was recently dubbed into Czech and is being used to train facilitators in the Czech Republic.

I was invited to contribute to the anthology *Voices on the Threshold of Tomorrow*, edited by Georg Feuerstein, Ph.D and Trisha Lamb Fuerstein. My chapter was entitled "Discovering and Recovering." The book was published by Quest Books in 1993.

My personal experience with co-dependence recovery was challenged to the utmost with a spouse with a chronic illness. I applied many of the learnings I shared in the original chapter. I, and we, continue to look for someone who knows more than we do in a particular area. We seek out information and are proactive in living with our challenges. We look for support, inspiration, and example in many areas.

One of the ways I found support for myself was by joining the Well Spouse Foundation. My "Declaration of Interdependence" was published in *MAINSTAY*, the September/October 1996 issue of the Foundation's Newsletter. The full title of my "Declaration" is "Help for the Well Spouse of a Person with Chronic Illness." My entrepreneurial spirit leads me to continue to share what I learn.

I would reiterate what I considered my most compelling learning in my original chapter "It's never too late to have a dream and follow it." Whatever my challenges, I can be gifted to grow through them if I remain congruent inside and outside and stay connected to the source of wisdom within.

Ann Marie Wyrsch
1360 South Fifth Street, Suite 390
St. Charles, MO 63301
(314) 947-0219

Chapter 27

Udderitis:
A Nursing Challenge

by Sharon A. Mathis, MPA, CRN, CNA

As I look back in retrospect over my nursing career, it was quite obvious that I would become an entrepreneur.

My background consisted of trying to help people who were less fortunate than I, as well as believing that all people are basically good. I took the role of patient advocate very seriously. I did not become a nurse to promote profits but to promote the well-being of patients.

My career as a nurse began in May of 1980 when I received my bachelor's degree in Nursing from Prairie View A & M University in Prairie View, Texas. I was a staff nurse and charge nurse during the years from 1980 through 1984. I practiced nursing in medical, surgical, and psychiatric settings in Houston. In 1984, I resigned my staff nurse position to accept my first management job as head nurse of a Dual Diagnosis Unit. One population was adolescent, and the other was young adults. It was a challenge for me to maintain these extremely different populations.

Within two years I was promoted to the director of the Adolescent Unit. Upon receiving this management job, I was also busy pursuing my master's degree in Public Administration. (I was learning daily that our profession was not respected as was the medical profession, and this was unacceptable to me.) I was always taught to plan ahead and not wait until a crisis occurred, therefore, I began to look at other career options

In May of 1987, I completed my MPA and decided it was time for another career move. The economy, the repeal of the Certificate of Need (hospitals no longer had to show a need for services to build a facility), hospital politics, and the closing of our unit motivated me to explore my options further. I left the corporation I was employed by to accept the challenge of a Director of Nursing position at another corporation. This was the best thing that could have happened to me and my entrepreneurial spirit.

In January of 1988 I began my new job. I was being surveyed by Medicare in April, JCAHO in November, and learning to adjust to new politics and a new community. The facility had not been surveyed under the new JCAHO standards, and its last survey had been three years earlier. I began "moving and shaking" to prepare for the tasks ahead of me.

During my tenure as Director of Nursing, I was faced with daily, weekly, and monthly challenges of full time equivalents, staff shortages, nursing care, and politics, politics, politics. I coined the word "udderitis" during my administration. An udder is the anatomical structure of the cow in which milk is expressed by pulling and pushing manually by the hands or milking machines. I felt this sensation on a day-to-day basis. I was always pulled in fifty million directions by personnel from all departments. As you know, nursing is the center of all activities within a hospital, and my inflamed udders were proof positive of this phenomenon.

Throughout my entire life I have always wanted to own my own business. My father inspired this through his entrepreneurship. I began looking very diligently at career alternatives for myself again.

184

I wanted to combine nursing with my administrative background.

I attended an annual nurse executive conference and was shocked at the high turnover of nurse executives. Attending another conference a month later uncovered additional information highlighting the shortage of nurse executives. I began to remember how overwhelming it was as a neophyte, as well as an experienced nurse executive.

I conducted a national search and could not find a company providing interim nurse managers/executives or support services. I asked myself, "Why are there support services for staff nurses, but none for nurse executives/managers?" I thought that it was ludicrous for the leaders of the profession not to have services which would allow them more time and energy to impact nursing practice and care daily.

Bells began to ring. What a concept! The shortage of nurses and the problems it creates impacted the turnover of nurse executives, as well as other variables. I really enjoyed nursing, but the lack of respect, creativity, control, and autonomy left a void in my professional career. My personal values were being challenged aggressively by politics. I had proven to myself that I could be a great director of nursing. However, I had other business, personal, and professional goals I wanted to achieve, therefore, I resigned my position as Director of Nursing and opened my own company.

Directions of Nursing Services (D.O.N.S.) was founded to provide interim nurse executives and managers, as well as offering consultations for healthcare facilities.

Nursing is forever standing at the crossroads of life—looking back over where we have been and looking ahead to where we will go. Our generation has a tough job. We must preserve our dreams in order that future generations will have life. So, with desire, determination, devotion, discipline, development and delivery, I challenge you to hold on to your dreams in order that we may share hope for the future.

UPDATE 1997

Although managed care has impacted my business goals, business is still booming!

We conduct health care expos—heath care community trade shows with seminars for health care professionals and community education for consumers. These are held in edifeces such as the summit (home of the back to back NBA Houston Rockets), the Houston Astrodome, and the George R. Brown Convention Center.

I write a monthly column for the *Houston Chronicle*—the largest newspaper in the southwest. I am also an advisory board member for its health care professional update publication.

We have added resources to service the home care industry. I am also a home care consultant. We assist individuals in starting home care agencies now known as home and community support agencies as well as develop strategies which keep them in business. We provide onsite and community education on home care topics for their employers and their staff.

In closing, time waits for no one. We must continue to achieve our dreams.

Directions of Nursing Services
6600 Hillcroft #2099
Houston, TX 77081
(713) 771-7043

Chapter 28

The Seed of the
Entrepreneurial Spirit

by Carolyn J. Taylor, P/MHNP

I was raised in a family that supported entrepreneurship, so it was in my blood to develop my own entrepreneurial spirit. After completing my graduate education and nurse practitioner certification, and with the state of Oregon being one of the first states to offer third-party reimbursement to nurse practitioners, it was natural that I would create a private practice.

My father lived on, and ran a farm, and was so productive that he was not allowed to be in the Army in World War I! He was rejected and told that he needed to stay home and raise food. He owned and developed two or three businesses in his lifetime, from plowing the ground for victory gardens during World War II to forming a successful electrical and plumbing business that he conducted until he was in his late seventies. The seed of my future business was planted in me as a child watching my father be successful in serving his community in the entrepreneurial spirit.

The seed started to germinate when I was the chairperson for the nursing program in a community college. It was becoming more evident that, as head of the department, I was spending more time doing crisis intervention and/or assisting students to deal with personal problems than I was spending in my commitment to preparing students to be effective nurses. I was becoming increasingly dissatisfied with working to keep an institutional structure in place—one that did not serve what I was committed to do.

After completing my graduate education and receiving my nurse practitioner certification, I decided to develop a private practice part-time. The first shoot broke ground. Third-party reimbursement for nurse practitioners had been passed in Oregon, so it seemed possible. While I was still administrating the Nursing program, I created a part-time office in our church and worked two evenings a week for a nominal fee.

Later, a friend who was also a nurse practitioner joined me, and we opened an office together. At that time I had to make a decision whether to open a full-time practice or to work at the college. I resigned from a tenured position, entered the partnership, and we opened The Wellness Place.

We received referrals from people we knew who had received value from our work with them. A family practice physician offered to refer patients to us if I would spend one day a week in his office. I agreed, and we raised our fees from $35 to $50 an hour. We became busier and more in demand.

Eventually, my partner chose not to spend her time and energy in the counseling profession and moved on to other avenues of expression, while I chose to remain in private practice. The change precipitated another raise in my fees so that I could hire a part-time secretary. My client list grew.

As the practice was expanding, my daughter, who was trained as a pediatric nurse, was noticing that working with sick children was increasingly harder for her to do. She had a desire to work with adults and chose to join me. We formed an entirely new business—Wellness Systems, Inc.—and set up an office in an athletic club in the heart of downtown. Just when our business was about to be in full bloom, its very existence was threatened.

We were set to complete whole-person assessments (physical, mental, emotional, social, and spiritual dimensions) and design programs for clients. In theory it was a wonderful vision, but we soon discovered that we were in over our heads:

1) We were in partnership with the wrong people;
2) We grew too big, too fast;
3) We were naive businesswomen;
4) Other people wanted too much cut into the business, and
5) We invested too much of our personal finances in the business.

We reached a point where we very nearly declared bankruptcy. Absolutely everything we owned was on the line. Could we save the business? What did we have to do to keep it alive?

True entrepreneurs that we were, we terminated unhealthy relationships, moved into a new office and created a new name for the business—The Taylor Group, Inc. We determined that we needed to practice what we practiced best—counseling, leading courses and training programs, and consulting to individuals, groups and organizations. We hired consultants ourselves, and we are now approaching the end of our 10th year of successful business at The Taylor Group, Inc. For the first several years, our gross income doubled on a yearly basis. We began with $9,900 in annual revenues, and the business will realize approximately $1 million for 1996.

Today, we work not only with private individuals and families, but with CEO's, company presidents, managers and their teams, many of who hold year-long contracts for consulting support. Additionally, we offer interventions in times of crisis such as natural disasters, unsolvable conflicts, or unexpected mergers, downsizing or other interruptions of work. We have three full-time counselors, one full time secretary, an executive assistant/office manager, and a chief financial officer and partner. In addition to working with people in and around our own metropolitan area, we counsel and work with people across the country via telephone and on-site visits.

The sudden death of my son eight years ago was a tragic event that affected each of us personally, profoundly and forever. For some, such an event would have proved the end of the business. Our own experience in facing and dealing with grief was in this case an unforeseen advantage, as we learned to maintain our focus and stability even while confronting personal tragedy and loss. We are, after all, well-being consultants, and we were able to use our knowledge in this area to assist ourselves in dealing with intense grief, and using that experience to develop courses that would serve others in similar circumstances.

Yes, my father would be proud of me, of us. We, too, have plowed a victory garden. The seed of the entrepreneurial spirit has grown and thrived, and continues to do so very successfully. We are feeding people a different kind of food—emotional and spiritual—and are carrying on the family tradition of service to the community.

The Taylor Group, Inc.
5520 S.W. Macadam Avenue, Suite 190
Portland, OR 97201
(503) 243-2846

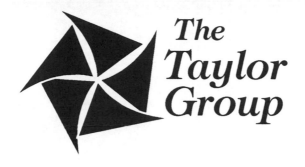

The Taylor Group

The Taylor Group

Well-being consultants for the health of people, their families, their enterprises.

Our Mission

To have people be well and productive.

Our Vision

Is for people of all generations to be effective in any circumstances encountered in life, freed of the past, and able to live joyfully and purposefully in the community while building a future for human spirit on the planet.

Our Work

Through a carefully designed process of questioning, clients begin to think and become more creative about the specific issues and concerns of their enterprises—particularly issues they thought had no probability of changing, or had nothing to do with them. Deeper structures of thinking and perception that shape the way people act are revealed. What is created is a possibility for being well, for being more effective with communication, relationships and life, and for having breakthroughs in performance and productivity.

5520 SW Macadam Ave.,Suite 190, Portland, Oregon 97201
Phone 503-243-2846   Fax 503-243-3635

Chapter 29

A Wake-Up Call To Action

by Clara E. Cornell, RN, MA

Sometimes it takes a wake-up call to spur me into action. I got that call just a year ago when I was negotiating to buy two companies. What started as an excellent relationship between the president of the companies and myself, as vice president, quickly turned sour as attorneys and accountants became involved.

For four years we had worked diligently to start five new healthcare companies in Pennsylvania. They were all doing well, so I approached the president with my offer to purchase two of them—a Medicare-certified home care and hospice agency and a professional medical brokerage firm.

We spent the next three months working with our respective "bean counters" and "mouthpieces." What do you think happened? They muddied that water! The time and money they were able to spend was incredible. I had no idea how much was involved with placing a value on a business. The president and I knew what the companies were worth and had already agreed upon a figure. Our "bean counters" thought differently. That was glitch #1.

Glitch #2 occurred with deciding appropriate dates for change of licensure. Believe me, choosing a date is somewhat like predicting when a baby will be born. Babies have ways of choosing their own dates—and they never seem to be at our convenience. Lawyers seem to operate in the same way. They want that baby to go to full term. It's better cash flow for them.

Glitch #3 came when we tried to divide the spoils, that is, divide payables and receivables. The last glitch—so I thought—was securing a bank loan and selecting the place for settlement.

Once all the details were ironed out and both camps were satisfied, we set the date for settlement. I breathed a sigh of relief. It wasn't until the night before settlement that I got my wake-up call. That's when the president told me she was not going to settle as planned. She wanted to postpone another month. Bells started going off in my head. Why cancel now, when the accountants and lawyers are all set? Did the other camp learn something that I didn't know? That wake-up call kept getting louder and louder. I responded as a true fighter—I ran! I called my attorney and said the baby wouldn't be born the next day. Instead, I decided to start my own company and forget the purchase.

My motivation for starting my own company came from this wake-up call. Looking back, I took an uncalculated risk that fortunately paid off. I made a decision to start only one of the companies— professional medical brokerage—in order to save money. Most of the staff followed, and are still with me. They sacrificed together with me to get the business started.

We opened our new office in a trailer occupied by three dogs. With wagging tails and barking mouths we greeted employees and customers with open arms. Furniture was all supplied by staff—kitchen tables, sewing machine cabinets, countertops on milk cartons, and cardboard box file cabinets. We tripped over each other to use the existing two phones. Many days I trotted out to my car in the snow and ice so I could use my car phone. At last, an open line. Two staff members were put out of the trailer to work out of their homes. They scheduled and interviewed and were accommodated with a one-person phone system.

Needless to say, this was a far cry from the luxurious offices we were accustomed to. We moved out when the fourth dog (and fleas) moved in. We opened a new office in one location—instead of three. We were equipped with a real Touch Tone office phone system and real office furniture.

The banker who was so willing to give me $250,000 suddenly gave me another wake-up call when he put obstacles in my path to secure a $50,000 line of credit, an amount documented in our business plan. That wake-up call was finally resolved when I got busy and refined the business plan for making the rounds for bank presentations.

I spent the next two weeks meeting bankers, educating them about medical brokerage of nurses to healthcare facilities, reviewing my business plan, and revealing all my personal assets. Finally, a young banker took an interest in my business and gave me the line of credit we needed. My wake-up call was finally in a position to pay off.

There were many sleepless nights spent wondering if payroll would be met for the 100 nurses who started with me at Health Staff, Inc. Those sleepless nights worrying about cash flow have now been re-placed by others. I now worry about new services we offer and whether we have the nurses to supply the needs of the facilities that call with their requests. Now we offer educational programs, certifi-cation workshops, home IV infusion, and permanent placement in addition to brokerage.

The wake-up call I received taught me many lessons. One lesson I learned was to be prepared for change. Change can happen at any time and most likely will happen when you don't expect it. Another lesson learned is that cash must be addressed before start-up. Just having a good idea is not enough. You must have sufficient working capital, and that is best demonstrated by a thorough and well-written business plan.

The absolute best lesson I learned is that *people* are so important. While all those wake-up calls were going off, my staff stuck by me. They sacrificed with me in the hard times, boosted my morale, and kept me on the right track. I could not have done it without them.

You better believe that wake-up call the night before settlement got my attention. But, you know what? I'm grateful!

HealthStaff, Inc.
P.O. Box 82
Dunmore, PA 18512
(717) 341-8200

Chapter 30

The Visionary Enterprise of Kind Hearts, Caring Hands

by Julia Cooper Oldfield, RN, BA

I keep seeing the commercial on TV that says something like, "If caring were enough, anybody could be a nurse." Well, caring isn't enough, that's for sure, but technical abilities and brains alone do not make a good nurse either. A good nurse has both, and she or he also cares. Sometimes too much—cares so much that often times she works overtime without being paid for it, volunteers to do double shifts even when her body says, "you're pushing me too hard," works wherever the healthcare facility sends her, even though she lacks the special skills to perform all the functions demanded of the assignment, thereby putting nursing licenses on the line.

I've been in those shoes I've described, and I have seen thousands of nurses in similar circumstances. I've known the frustration of being so short staffed that I felt guilty, because it seemed that I had little time for nurturing, and just barely enough time to pass meds, give baths, change dressings, check IV's, and chart.

What does this have to do with my becoming a nurse entrepreneur? I decided that being a good nurse meant taking good care of myself as well as my patients. This decision was practically forced on me as I began to suffer a variety of injuries beginning in 1980—first, a severe lumbar sprain and then a couple of years later, a brachial plexus nerve entrapment. I endured periods of severe pain, surgery, and long episodes of rehabilitation. It was during these times that I began to learn I had to take care of myself, and that taking pills and having surgery weren't the only ways to heal myself.

Hence, my journey toward becoming a nurse entrepreneur began first toward healing and helping myself, and eventually working with others to do the same. I spent months in severe pain, in physical therapy, on muscle relaxants, and learning what the role of the patient was about. Helpless and hopeless at times, I felt despair and depression. Then I started a journey within, a journey toward healing and hope.

First, I began reading all I could on various holistic healing methods and learned to use biofeedback for pain control, which was very successful. I also used music therapy, meditation, and positive affirmations. My bathroom mirror was covered by little cards with such statements as: *I am vitally alive and radiantly beautiful, I take good care of myself, I am healthy, strong and happy,* and, *I am directed to my highest good and the good of all.*

My health made a remarkable recovery, and I eventually, went to work for a major medical malpractice insurance carrier as a risk management consultant representing healthcare facilities nationwide. This prestigious position put me in consultation on a daily basis with hospital administrators, directors of nursing, department managers, and hospital staffs. I also taught literally hundreds of classes on quality assurance and risk management issues. I worked with, and observed the circumstances, morale, and conditions of American healthcare professionals. I found that my earlier experiences as a hospital nurse were common among those I observed, and I saw a need for nurturing the nurturers and providing opportunities for them to learn skills which they could use, not only for themselves, but also to teach to their patients.

As a result of a compelling drive to discover how I could best help fill this need and fulfill myself, I left my position with the insurance company in 1988 and decided to give myself some time to allow my ideas and direction to form. I continued to study and practice holistic healing modalities. From 1984 to 1986, I had attended college while working full-time to complete a BA degree, majoring in Psychology. Drawing upon my nursing experiences gained in positions in coronary care, med-surg, pediatric office nursing, QA, UR, mental health, chemical dependence, rehab, infection control, and education, I considered the various options and directions open to me.

In 1990, I formed Visionary Enterprises, Inc., and a division of that corporation is Kind Hearts, Caring Hands, a name that came to me in an early morning dream-like state, while I was recuperating from an auto accident. Kind Hearts, Caring Hands provides healthcare consulting and education to nurses and the general public. Our focus is on what I call "adjuncts to medical and psychological interventions," fancy words which simply mean methods to help the person enhance the healing process. We offer individualized stress management programs, reflexology, music as a healing modality, aromatherapy, therapeutic touch, guided imagery, and hypnosis, as well as career counseling. I provide private sessions in some of these areas and utilize the services of independent practitioners in others. We are also planning to include classes on image and communication skills as well as risk management education programs on our 1991-92 calendar. Being aware of your personal responsibility and liability is another way of taking good care of yourself.

I utilized the services of a marketing consultant and an attorney/CPA from the onset of my business, and interviewed a number of consultants before I began planning my first seminar. My office is in my home, and I have a separate telephone number for the business. I have utilized secretarial services on a project basis, as I am not yet in a position to employ a secretary, nor do I need one on a daily basis. I have created most of the handout materials myself on our computer— an absolute must for a business, not a luxury by any means. The capital I used to start the business came from personal funds. I must say, the costs for the first year were well beyond my projections. If I could go back to the beginning, I think I would have arranged a business loan rather than use personal funds.

Nonetheless, I am pleased with the planning and preparation taken to form and implement my business. For the first year, I have planned to present quarterly seminars and publish quarterly newsletters. The first newsletter was distributed in October of 1990, and the first seminar was in November of 1990. The response was very favorable.

I have developed a polished, professional, quality product which I am proud of. There is no profit yet, but with less than a year in operation, that is not expected. Part of planning a successful business is knowing how fast you can afford to grow. The interest expressed has reinforced my belief that there is a need for these services, and that those people who want to help themselves and others will utilize us as a learning resource as they become more aware of what we offer.

If I could write a commercial for my philosophy, it would say, "Nurturing yourself nurtures others. If you care for others, take care of yourself."

UPDATE 1997

Kind Hearts, Caring Hands was a labor of love. I poured a lot of heart, time, and money into the venture, but in 1992, had to set it aside to go back to work for a large healthcare corporation which could provide me with a regular salary and benefits. I still believe in the concept of my business, but timing is everything, "they say," and I think my timing was off. The recession which impacted *me* really began in 1989, and by 1992, I could no longer afford to keep putting money into my business without getting enough from it to at least pay its operating costs.

Healthcare delivery systems also began a dramatic change in the way they provided education opportunities for nurses. Many healthcare settings laid off their education department staffs and stopped all but the state-required continuing education classes for their nurses. Hospitals sharply reduced their inpatient beds and staffs as well. Nurses were often left to find their own avenues for meeting continuing education requirements, with no financial support from their employers. This impacted my business.

Becoming a nurse entrepreneur was a wonderful experience. I learned a great deal, made new friends, and provided a service for the benefit of those I hold in high esteem, healthcare professionals. Now, more than ever before, the type of services Kind Hearts, Caring Hands provided, as well as the philosophy behind it, are needed. "To be the best nurse you can be, you must first be kind and caring to yourself. When the vessel is empty, what can come from it?"

Kind Hearts, Caring Hands
10153 1/2 Riverside Drive, Suite 588
Toluca Lake, CA 91602
(818) 509-WELL

A Division of Visionary Enterprises, Inc.

Chapter 31

You Only Go This Way Once

by Patricia W. Iyer, RN, MSN, CNA

Imagine the scene: you're six months pregnant with your second child when your husband's business fails.

He borrowed $1 million to start a business in the early 1980s, including $20,000 from your mother. For five years he worked seven days a week, twelve hours a day, but could not make the business successful. Your marriage is still intact, although your first child hardly knows his father. At the end of five years, when he's had to close down the business, the lenders are circling your house like sharks.

In the midst of your pregnancy the bank is getting assessments of your house to see if it's worth taking to satisfy some of your debt load. (After all, you both signed a personal guarantee agreeing to surrender all of your assets if you reneged on the business loan payments.) Your mother decides she wants her money repaid now, when you have almost no income from the business. Your husband, who has finely honed his bargaining skills, negotiates a way to satisfy some of the debts so you can keep your personal assets. He does not have to declare bankruptcy. You cash in your IRA's and pay back your mother, but it takes a year before the relationship with her heals.

Why would anyone who has gone through something like this want to start a business? And what lessons would you learn from that experience? The pregnant wife in the above story was me—now president of two businesses, mother of two, and still married to the same entrepreneurial husband.

How did we pick up the pieces? My second son was born in 1983. At that time I was working in an acute-care hospital as director of the Staff Development Department. I liked my job and had no plans to leave. My husband began a brokering business in our home after walking away from the ashes of his dreams. (His business is now stable and growing.)

The first step toward opening the door of my own business started in 1982, when I co-authored a self-learning module on the nursing process. It was used to teach the nurses in my facility about nursing diagnosis. My two co-authors and I decided to submit the module to publishers. The first publisher who responded said that we should expand the module into a textbook, and that it could not be sold as written. "That's too much work," we said, and continued to try other publishers. When the second publisher gave us the same advice, we decided to listen.

The publication of *Nursing Process and Nursing Diagnosis* by W.B. Saunders in 1986 opened the door to opportunities by establishing my credentials as an expert in the nursing process. I had visions of gaining professional recognition for my accomplishment, but I found that a prophet in his own land is not always acknowledged. Some of the nurses I worked with at the hospital congratulated me on the publication of the book, but others said, "It's only Pat Iyer. I don't know what all the fuss is about." I sensed that I needed to move beyond my job in order to build on the processes set in motion by the publication of the book.

Six months after the book came out, I left my job where I'd worked for seven years and took a new job at a different hospital as a nursing quality assurance coordinator. This was the transition step that I needed to wrench myself away from the comforting environment where I'd spent seven years. I moved from education to quality assurance because of a perception that skills in QA would be marketable. The task of creating a QA program out of nothing was exciting. However, what I did not foresee was the effects of commuting to the job. I drove more than an hour on heavily traveled roads with tractor trailers who liked to play bumper tag. While I got up at 5:30 a.m. and was ready for sleep by 9:00 p.m., the rest of my family was on a different time schedule and resented mine. After several months it was clear to me that the hospital was not going to move any closer to me, and I had no desire to leave our home in a rural environment and move my family closer to the job.

While I was trying to find a way out of my dilemma, I attended a seminar on career choices that pushed me the rest of the way through the door of opportunity and motivated me to take the plunge. I reached one decision very early in the planning process. I would not involve myself in any business that involved borrowing money. All of a sudden I realized that I could put bits and pieces together to form a business. My husband's business was doing well, and I had the luxury to take a risk. Before I resigned my job, I had an interview with my former boss and discussed consulting services that I could offer. She expressed interest, and on the strength of her positive response, I left my job in November of 1987. I took a month-long trip to India with my family, and returned to open the doors of Patricia Iyer Associates.

When I stepped through the threshold into the new world of being an independent businesswoman, I took a long look at my assets and capabilities. My list of strengths included a master's degree in Nursing, certification in nursing administration, current knowledge of acute-care nursing and quality assurance, teaching and writing skills, a network of professional acquaintances, a good relationship with a major publisher, and low overhead expenses.

My main drawback was the fact that I disliked selling myself, my services, and products. After thinking about the various ways in which I could earn money, and reaffirming that I did not want to take on the expenses of an office, I got some letterhead printed and set about marketing my skills. In the first year and a half I earned money from the following sources: weekend staff nursing; royalties from my first book, and then from the second one which was published in 1989, *Nursing Diagnosis and Care Planning* (W.B.Saunders); expert witness review of nursing malpractice cases; teaching seminars on nursing diagnosis, documentation and quality assurance as a subcontractor for other nurse entrepreneurs and a national seminar company; consulting in quality assurance; and reviewing manuscripts for nursing publishers.

I was rolling along this path, feeling increasingly more secure and fulfilled, when one day in 1989 I got a phone call. The attorney who was calling wanted me to review a case involving a plaintiff who was injured in an Emergency Department. I explained that I had no ED background, but gave him the name of one of my acquaintances who was an ED clinical specialist. When he thanked me and contacted the specialist, the light bulb went off in my brain. I realized that there was money to make by providing a referral service for malpractice attorneys looking for expert witnesses. Med League Support Services was born in April of 1989. I attended an excellent seminar and learned the variety of services that could be offered in a medical-legal support business. This branch of my activities involves providing services to malpractice attorneys, including screening cases for merit, helping to organize records, and referrals of expert witnesses. To date, most of my requests for help come from attorneys looking for experts.

Having discovered that publishing is part of the key to establishing credentials as an expert, in 1989 I was ready to embark upon my third book. I co-authored this book with a nurse I had met through teaching for the national seminar company. *Nursing Documentation, a Nursing Process Approach* was published by Mosby Year Book in 1991. It is a product of three years of teaching about nursing documentation in the U.S. and Canada, countless hours spent reading nursing literature on documentation, and the lessons I'd learned from being an expert witness, The publication of this book established my expertise in documentation and nursing liability.

By early 1990, I'd been on the road for three years teaching programs all over the U.S and Canada, learning how to navigate around airports and sleep in strange hotel beds. While I enjoyed traveling, my family did not enjoy having me gone for a few days at a time and made their feelings clear. In addition, the seminar company for whom I worked did not permit me to market my services at the programs I taught for them. I began to perceive that the programs were dead ends from a marketing perspective, so I started to consider other alternatives.

While I was wallowing in indecision and self-doubt, I connected with another nurse entrepreneur who encouraged me to cut loose from the seminar company and to recognize that I had very marketable skills. If I was spending time and money marketing my own services, why not be able to offer a greater variety of services by hooking up with other experts? Patricia Iyer Associates expanded in early 1990 to included three additional nurses: a management educator/consultant, a critical care educator, and a computer consultant. As president of this group, I market our services through networking and direct mail.

I've also developed a line of audiotapes on a variety of subjects. Although I have recorded some of these tapes, a greater number have been recorded for me by a variety of experts. Based on my experiences as a writer receiving royalties from publishing companies of anywhere from 10-15 percent, I decided to give my authors 50 percent royalties from sales of the tapes. It is exciting to watch the line of tapes grow as I network and reach out to nurses with expertise in specific areas. For a person who hated to sell, I have learned to market my tapes through direct mail, distributorship arrangements, and catalogs. In 1990, Patricia Iyer Associates became the first nurse-owned business in my state to be an approved provider of continuing education. Therefore, I can offer contact hours for my in-house seminars and audiotapes.

As I look ahead to the future, I envision growth in the line of audiotapes, new distributorship arrangements, increased use of my associates' expertise, increased use of networking as a marketing strategy for building my businesses, and expansion of my medical-legal business. I look forward to new opportunities to grow, and would be very hard pressed to return to being an employee.

The following are some random thoughts for aspiring entrepreneurs who may benefit from some of the lessons I've learned the hard way: Don't borrow money to start a business if you can possibly avoid it, and never borrow money from relatives or friends.

Keep your overhead low in the beginning. Work out of your home, if possible, and learn to say, "My office is in (name of town)," or "I won't be in my office tomorrow." You don't have to advertise the fact that you work out of your house. Be sure you have self-discipline when operating from your home office. Some entrepreneurs complain that they have trouble avoiding distractions when they need to be working. Others, like myself and my husband, have difficulty turning the work off at the end of the day and find ourselves working into the evening and weekends. Be sure to block off time to spend with your family.

Don't overlook the power of establishing your credentials by writing for publication. Start with articles before tackling a book, and ask someone with writing skills to help organize and edit your manuscript before submitting it.

Think carefully before investing in an expensive brochure and mass mailings. Although I have done both, I have found that mass mailings were not nearly as effective as I hoped they would be. If you use your children to help assemble business literature, pay them by the piece, not by the hour. When my highly-intelligent older son assembled brochures, his productivity declined with time. Monotonous work like copying and stuffing envelopes can be taken only in small doses.

Network with other nurse entrepreneurs, potential clients, and anyone you think will help pass on the word about your business. If someone's referral helps you land a job, send a thank-you note to the person who gave your name.

Remember that the nursing community is a small one. Try not to do or say anything that will come back to haunt you later.

Consider brushing up on your clinical skills so that you are able to work on a per diem basis. My occasional role as a staff nurse provides me with great rewards— increased credibility as an expert witness, or, when I teach, an easy way to earn money during low income times, and the satisfaction of helping patients.

Don't be afraid to ask questions, ask for help, or learn and grow.

You only go this way once, and you should spend your life doing something you enjoy.

UPDATE 1997

The five years since the first edition of this book have flown by. After reviewing the original chapter, I realized how the focus of my business has narrowed. Forces that have reshaped healthcare directed my attention away from teaching nurses and consulting with hospitals. Four years ago, as enrollments declined in the continuing education market, and hospitals cut back on money available for consultants, I recognized that I needed to change the thrust of my business. Since I had no desire to return to an employee status, I again looked at my business with a critical eye. This is what I found: My review of cases as an expert witness was satisfying and resulted in carrying over the risk prevention principles into my teaching and consulting. Expert witness work also whetted my appetite to expand my medical legal business. I began actively marketing and building a support business for attorneys. I found a market that was somewhat uninformed about how a nurse could help in personal injury cases. However, once an attorney understands the benefits of working with a nurse, it is usually much easier to develop an ongoing business relationship.

My medical legal support business has gradually expanded to limit the amount of attention that can be paid to other business activities. While it was important in the beginning to have a broad focus, I was forced to concentrate on one business rather than keep several ones functioning. With the expansion of my consulting business, my staff increased to two and one half full time secretaries, a nurse and a dozen nursing subcontractors. This has also necessitated moving the business out of our home and into an office environment. All of this has been accomplished without borrowing a dime. The specter of bankruptcy is not easily forgotten.

I would like to add to the advice to aspiring entrepreneurs that ended the previous version of this chapter.

Don't be afraid to reach out and call nurses who are in business to ask specific, targeted questions. If they suggest that you send them information, such as your resume, do follow through.

A good computer system and a separate phone line from the household line are essential for establishing a professional image. Avoid call waiting if possible, as many people are finding it increasingly annoying. It is better to invest in a separate line that is attached to an answering machine to take a call when you cannot do so.

Learn as much as you can about the business you wish to enter. Do not overlook the knowledge that can be gained by buying books, taking courses and finding people who can help you get started.

There are few overnight successes. Do not lose heart or motivation if the business is slow in getting started.

As your business grows, recognize that it is easy to lose sight of the need to relax and take time off. When you find that every waking hour is being spent on the business, it is time to loosen the reins, bring in a partner, employee or otherwise find a way to reclaim your leisure time. Burnout can reduce the motivation of nurse entrepreneurs and take some of the joy out of owning business. Keep in mind that when you own a business, you should enjoy the benefits and fruits of your labor without letting the business own you.

Patricia Iyer Associates
55 Britton Road, Suite 500
Stockton, NJ 08559
(908) 788-8227

Chapter 32

Chicken Soup
And What?

by Mary M. Baker, RNC, MHS, FNP

It was 3 a.m.—my room was spinning—*true vertigo!* A textbook classic—why me? Why now? The year was 1980; the month, September. A month I'll never forget. I was working with a physician specializing in geriatrics and internal medicine. Yes, I knew exactly what I had—the etiology was either viral or bacterial, and I knew that Antivert would stop the room from spinning in circles and discontinue the dizziness and nausea—then perhaps I could lift my head from the pillow...

Later that day, once I got the Antivert into my system and experienced my "sea legs," I began to think. If I got so ill this fast, could diagnose myself, but couldn't do a damn thing to assist myself—how many folks out there were in need of TLC, home care, practical advice, and therapeutic nursing intervention? The need was becoming self-evident, the idea was taking shape.

When I was back on my feet again I talked to my physician colleague. Being a single woman, I was feeling and understanding the need for an investment in my future. The law had just changed in California. Registered nurses could now own up to 49 percent of a medical practice. I wanted to invest in the practice. I was a cost-effective nurse practitioner building a practice.

My esteemed colleague told me that incorporating was like getting married. I was astounded. "Yes," I said, "it was a legal contractual relationship, but I somehow feel that marriage *is* slightly different." He chewed on his handle bar mustache, then said, "Perhaps it is, but I am not interested in incorporating at this time."

"Okay. I need to invest in my future. Building your practice does not do that for me. I guess I need to look for an opportunity that will."

At that point, I was feeling discouraged. I started thinking of leaving nursing. Go into business! Yes, there was opportunity in business. What kind? Well, I didn't know, but there had to be more than continuing as a nurse practitioner building a physician's practice. I discussed the plan with a friend and mentor who had supervised a work project in business while I had been in graduate school. He firmly stood his ground. "Think creatively! You are so good at what you do. You've worked hard to get there—don't change horses in midstream—*think creatively!*"

A period of three or four months passed. The memory of the vertigo, the dizziness of making a career change, the feeling of helplessness, my love of public health/community nursing kept humming in the back of my mind. "*Think creatively!*" was ever-present on my mind. Externally, I was talking the I-have-to-leave-nursing litany to make the knock of opportunity succeed. Business. The answer was going into business.

At some point the idea for a home nursing service for normally healthy people who had a short-term illness (like me) just seemed right. A new option on the spectrum of healthcare choices. I'd never heard of anything like it. I had worked for a Visiting Nurse Association in the past. The healthy adult with an acute illness would never contemplate calling a Visiting Nurse Association for assistance. I wouldn't. The light bulb went off. The ahahhhhhaa experience occurred. The germinal idea had taken shape.

From that point on, I wrote down every facet of the proposed service that occurred to me. I talked to friends and non-nursing associates in the community. I later found out that I had done an informal marketing survey. I kept revising, revamping, and re-evaluating the concept in writing. I discussed the project with my mentor. He encouraged me. It made sense to him. He had been in business for fifty years. He was not a healthcare professional, but he did know people, the marketplace, and (most essentially) the community.

I quit my full-time job with the mustachioed M.D. I accepted a job with a pulmonary and infectious disease group working as a practitioner twenty hours a week. This part-time status allowed me to continue developing the concept and finance my living expenses. When friends got sick, I would make a house call and do the assessment. The prototype of the service was perfected.

Finally, in August of 1981, I sent out my press releases. Chicken Soup, Plus. The Home Nursing Service & Nursing Practice was formed. I had thought of the name Chicken Soup. The connotations of TLC and personalized care communicated my philosophy. My friend and mentor added the *Plus*, saying, "You will be doing more than you think—providing services that you can't even imagine at this point in time." So, Chicken Soup, Plus it was. The response from the media to the press release was overwhelming. Radio talk shows, news items in the newspaper, and TV interviews—they all wanted to go on a house call.

We are currently in our tenth year of business. During five of those years, we had a family practice clinic in the office as well as the home nursing service. It was stressful dealing with third-party payors. They pay very slowly. Overhead is constant and demanding. We had a family practice physician and one to three other nurse practitioners seeing patients four half-days per week. Insurance billing, balancing the budget, watching cash flow, and marketing were concepts that were new to me, even though as a nurse practitioner, cost-effective services and collections were second nature. I embellished the skills I had and developed and identified new areas of strength and interest.

Today, my company is a California corporation. We have had a service mark registered with the Federal Government and the Secretary of the State of California since April of 1981. We specialize in respite care staffing in the consumer's home. We also provide case management consultation and services. We continue to offer home nursing visits to new moms, adults with elimination management difficulties, and acutely-ill children. We have contracts with groups to provide pre-employment physical exams, assessments of ADL (activities of daily living), and make recommendations to the housing authority in regard to client suitability and level of care needed.

I do consulting and national speaking on ethics, running a business, marketing, future trends, and strategic planning. I was recently asked to contribute an article for the December 1990 issue of the *Nurse Practitioner Forum*, celebrating the 25th anniversary of nurse practitioners. I see that writing and publishing are two important areas of development for me in the future.

The lessons I have learned are many. The hardest was middle-management delegation. The most important is to *think creatively*! Even if the idea or dream is not present in the marketplace, as you develop the concept branches and leaves will appear from the initial germinal idea. Among the other pearls that I have gleaned in these past ten years are the following:

1. See frustration as a challenge
2. Become known as an expert in your community
3. Always commit your ideas to paper
4. Necessity *is* the mother of invention. Just because you can't do everything needed in running a business, don't underestimate

your capabilities to learn or to get help.

5. Do not see "failure" as an end—perhaps it is the beginning of an even better idea.
6. Consider creating an advisory committee of people whose opinions and business acumen you respect.
7. Always see the consumer as your #1 strategic partner in any venture.

So, from the vertigo I experienced initially, to the "dizzy" life of an entrepreneur—the situations are not so far afield, are they?

UPDATE 1997

Many exciting things have been happening since the original publication of the story of this nurse entrepreneur. Chicken Soup, Plus, The California Corporation, expanded to include a Medicare division providing the complete selection of professional, skilled intermittant services: skilled nursing, the therapies (physical, speech, occupational, medical social work) as well as home health aide and dietician care.

Due to the configuration requirements and oversight of the government, it became very apparent that I needed to separate the Medicare Division from the long standing traditional continuous home care and (now—new buzz word) managed care line of services. As of January 1, 1995 two separate corporations were established—Chicken Soup, Plus, The California Corporation providing continuous and Managed Home Care, and Chicken Soup, Plus., Home Health Care Incorporated providing the Medicare, Medicaid home health care.
In July of 1994, the marketplace of healthcare was in an accelerated condition of deregulation. Sacramento, in particular was/is a bee-hive of Managed Care activity. Over 90% of people in Sacramento are covered by an HMO or managed by their employer health plans. I

217

am not sure of the statistic statewide, but shall we suffice it to say—California is one of the managed care hot beds! Now—how were we nurse entrepreneurs going to survive? There was no national model for nursing's response. I convened a group of 10 nurse entre-executives in home healthcare. The group formed a cohesive unit and by December 1994 were incorporated as National Independent Nursing Network, the first IPA owned and operated by registered nurses. The purpose of the group was survival in the managed care arena—to enter into statewide (and eventually, national) contracts with other IPA's, PPO's, HMO's and insurance companies to provide home healthcare.

We represented geographically the entire state. I (as founder) was elected as the President of the Corporation. By February 1995 we hired an Executive Director and also a registered nurse, established an office in Sacramento and headed out to develop a network and get contracts.

Here we are two years later - with California coverage - 35-37 sites of licensed and certified home health care in California. Statewide contracts centralized billing and collections. The NINN is not a profitable venture as yet. We are currently at a turning point. The rearranged care market is rapidly evolving. We constantly strategize how to meet the market demands.

Developing a viable operation with a working board of nurse entrepreneurs has been a challenge. We have all shared, grown, developed our businesses and friendships, and inspiring colleagealities that will help us and our businesses in the future.

Chicken Soup, Plus.—both Corporations—continue to flourish. I am considering the purchase of commercial real estate for the Medicare Division, and expect JACHO to have accreditted us by the end of 1996.

Where are Medicare, managed care and healthcare going as we approach the next century? I am not certain; however I do know that running a "lean machine" these days is critical to the financial viability of any and all operations. It is essential that we all carry on with excitement, dedication, creativity and renewed faith in ourselves—as nurse entrepreneurs, as patient advocates, as business people, alert and aware of the shifts occurring in the paradigm and the market place. We must continue to contribute and make a difference and above all support other Nurses in Business!

Chicken Soup, Plus
1725 10th Street
Sacramento, CA 95814
(916)443-6429

Chapter 33

Flight of the Dove

by Sarah A. Seybold, RN, MSM

When my partner Barbara O'Reilly was ten years old, she was a mid-western 4-H member already sewing her own clothes. At half that age I was ringing Southern California neighborhood doorbells, selling songs (singing in pig-Latin was five cents extra). By the age of ten I'd sold misletoe, child care, a dogwalking service, and flowers—never mind where I got them. Many years before we met, Barbara and I were already developing the skills that made us believe we could get Dove to fly.

Dove Professional Apparel was named for the symbol of peace and hope, and began in a fever of idealism. The three of us who started the company were among the founders of the San Francisco-based Center for US-USSR initiatives, and we hoped Dove would support us so we could continue building bridges of peace and friendship between the citizens of the United States and the Soviet Union.

At the end of the 1983 school year, I met Sharon Tennison, the mother of one of my university nursing students. She was an ICU nurse who, as a member of Physicians for Social Responsibility, had been speaking to church and civic groups about the global threat of nuclear war. The question "What about the Russians?" came again and again from her audiences, so she had determined to meet "the enemy" face to face. I came home the night of my first meeting with Sharon and announced, to my husband's amazement, that I was going on a peace mission to the Soviet Union!

Barbara O'Reilly was also among the twenty-three professional people on that first trip at the height of the Cold War, only a few weeks after Korean Airlines flight 007 was shot down. As citizen-diplomats we spoke at church and civic forums after the trip and helped to establish the Center, which has become a leading organization for citizen-initiated exchanges between Soviets and Americans.

But citizen diplomacy was full-time involvement. I had left my teaching position and Sharon, the Center's director, had no time for ICU work. How to pay our bills?

The answer, we thought, was stored in Sharon's garage—the remaining inventory of a uniform business she had started in 1981 and put on hold. Sharon had grown up in the South, and like Barbara, had developed her sewing talents. She had invented a nursing apron with unique sectioned pockets that allowed her to carry needed supplies and instruments, providing organization that increased her efficiency in the ICU and on hospital floors. Other nurses deluged her with requests for similar aprons with pockets. Then nurses suggested putting sectioned pockets on dresses and jackets. When Sharon could no longer handle the sewing, she hired a skilled seamstress.

Sharon's business was still on hold in 1983, but Barbara and I seemed to provide the elements needed to revive it. Barbara, a home economics teacher with experience in small business, had begun in childhood to develop her specialty in textiles. And I had never lost my childhood flair for sales, which had only been enhanced by fifteen years in nursing education.

I knew firsthand the problems nursing students had with professional image and their dissatisfaction with traditional student uniforms, and I saw my nursing education experience as a direction for our company.

There followed lean years of anxious marketing calls, lugging boxes of nursing uniforms, teetering on the brink of success, of failure and exhaustion. Barbara began the tedious task of resizing and standardizing the patterns. With our miniscule budget, we agonized over advertising, artwork, taking out loans, and reserving convention space.

But Dove uniforms have made a hit. We have a quality product that nurses appreciate and a file of testimonials praising our quality fabric, designs, attentive service, and the unique pockets with the Dove trademark. The acceptance has kept us going. At nursing conventions, ours is often the busiest booth—on several occasions reps from other companies have asked to be hired by Dove.

Starting a business has been like winding up a toy that takes off down the path, leaving you breathless trying to catch up.

At first we rode off in all directions, setting up displays and toting the inventory anywhere we thought we might make a sale. I once sat with my uniforms in an empty patient room at Saint Mary's Hospital at 3 a.m., hoping to find new customers among the night nurses. Getting a hospital to agree to a sale of nursing uniforms was a major accomplishment. There were frustrations and rejections. But a couple of former colleagues put in a good word for us, and a nun who taught me in nursing school opened a key hospital door.

In those early days we had the energy and enthusiasm—and naivete—related to a new hobby. We hooted with delight when we had a week's gross receipts of $250!

Our first break was the contract to provide uniforms for all of the student nurses at Gavilan College. Faculty and student committees chose Dove as the required uniform. That success confirmed the marketing direction that has carried us into the black and has actually allowed us to pay ourselves a salary—still small, but increasing. We now have seventeen nursing school contracts, and we acquire new ones each semester.

Perhaps our biggest accomplishment is our recent joint venture agreement with the American Nurses Association, which created a mail-order catalog of products for nurses. The agreement provides that ANA will advertise our products to its 200,000 members at a 10 percent discount. The response has been exhilarating.

The experience of launching Dove has taught us to grow the business gradually. Steady is best. But perhaps it's more accurate to say that the business grows *us*. We have acquired skills roughly at a pace with the expansion of our company. Barbara and I have become Macintosh afficianados of a sort. And we have a seat-of-the-pants mastery of basic marketing, graphics, shipping, banking, finance, accounting, and taxes. Necessity is the mother of improvisation as well as invention.

Business people will not be surprised to learn that Dove has become our full-time occupation (except for Sharon, who remains the administrator of the Center for US-USSR Initiatives and has now traveled to the Soviet Union more than thirty times).

Advice to nurses hoping to succeed in business? First of all, love your product or service; be utterly sold on its value and validity. Next, become computer literate—or befriend a dataprocessing whiz (how did businesses ever exist without computers?). A large percentage of small businesses fold within their first few years, the majority because of undercapitalization and the inability to handle information. Finally, don't expect to be rolling in money overnight. First you have to pay your dues. Fortunately, we both had support from our husbands, who made it possible for us to work at very low wages.

We're still paying our dues. You should see us in our makeshift office, what we refer to as corporate headquarters, or in the "Dove Coop," the tiny cottage where we warehouse our inventory. The situation is temporary—we will grow one step at a time.

In spite of the frustrations and trials of a small start-up company, we have maintained a great deal of our idealism. We strive toward a model of ethical business and are committed to respect for the environment and to our motto: *Nurses helping nurses with image and organization.*

We're confident Dove will soar. Remember, the dove is a symbol of hope.

UPDATE 1997

Five years after the publication of "Flight of the Dove" my partner and I are still fluttering our wings with lusty vigor. Dove Professional Apparel has grown steadily at the healthy rate of more than twenty percent a year. July of 1996 was the biggest revenue month in Dove's history. In our peak season we have no difficulty keeping ten employees busy in our office, with another ten or fifteen at the manufacturing site. We have half a dozen representatives ready to do fittings and take orders at many of the eighty colleges we now serve.

If Dove's employees were to visit our original office space, Barbara's garage, it would look like a 1960s telephone booth stuffing contest. We have moved twice in the last five years, like a teenager growing out of his shoes. Our current space is commodious and pleasant, with room on the floor for our daily abdominal and back strengthening class for all employees.

Dove has been lucky, but we have provided much of own luck. We see it in our employees. A retired school teacher has been with us since the garage days. Our accountant came out of retirement because he admired our spunk and style and wanted to help Dove grow. The younger half of the staff is a corps of high school and college girls who are maturing before our eyes, and grace the company with their vivacity and dedication. They conduct telephone business with remarkable skill. We have committed ourselves to enlightened personnel policies to maximize for both the company and the employees the benefits of working at Dove. We offer a paid retreat day each year to every employee; we have company picnics and trips to the movies, and the daily thirty-minute "abs" class, led by our newest employee, who is also a chiropractor.

Dove prides itself on quality of product and quality of service. Often we have won a new college contract in the same area as an existing one, because a clinical nursing instructor has seen students from another school in Dove uniforms. Our garments and our reputation for service help to market Dove. Perhaps unique in the industry is the publication, in the neck label of each garment, of our 800 telephone number. Many nurses have been able to refer colleagues to us immediately when their uniforms or lab coats have been admired. The 800 number on the label has been a risk as a boon, since it also brings us face to face with an occasional customer complaint. But we are resolved to handle all calls with courtesy and care. It is work for our souls, we remind ourselves, as well as for our profits. My daughter, who works at a giant corporation, admires the relaxed and nurturing atmosphere at Dove, in contrast to the pressure and tension at her workplace.

Barbara and I look back on the decade or so of our partnership with satisfaction and pride. As we approach retirement, we are trying to build Dove to the point where it will be irresitible to potential buyers. Our dream is to pass on the enterprise to other nurses, whose training and philosophy will carry on the spirit of Dove's flight.

Dove Professional Apparel
663 Bernardo #B-1
Sunnyvale, CA 94087
(415) 968-DOVE

AT LAST!

A User-Friendly Uniform for the Health Care Professional

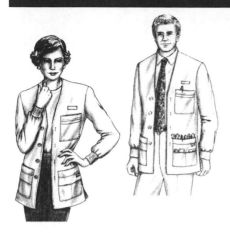

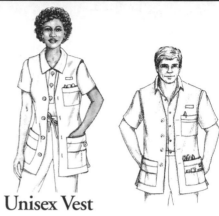

Unisex Vest

P, S, M, L, XL, XXL ($39), XXXL ($44)
Jacket length, upper pocket, inner pocket with velcro closure, nametag holder, side vents.
White, Navy or Light blue.

V-Neck Cardigan (Unisex)

P, S, M, L, XL, XXL ($44), XXXL ($49)
Push-up sleeves with knit cuffs, side vents, inner pocket with velcro closure, upper pocket, name pin holder. White, Navy or Light blue.

CALL TOLL-FREE
1-800-829-3683

Quantity	Size	Color	Description	Price

Dove Professional Apparel
1674 N. Shoreline Blvd., Suite A-1
Mountain View, CA 94043-1316

sub total	
applicable tax*	
shipping/ins.	$6.00
TOTAL	

* CA residents, please add tax for your counties.

___ A check for amount due is enclosed

___ Charge my Visa/Masatercard ☐☐☐☐☐☐☐☐☐☐☐☐☐☐☐☐☐☐☐☐

    Signature _____ Exp. Date _____

___ Please send brochure of all styles.

Name _____

Address _____

City _____ Zip _____ Tel. _____

America's Freedom Fabric
VISA BY M LIKEN
America's Freedom Fabric

■ PLEASE SEND INFORMATION ABOUT THE PURCHASE OF A DOVE FRANCHISE

Chapter 34

Expanding Nursing Frontiers

(This profile appeared in the November 1988 issue of the *Nurse-Entrepreneur's Exchange.*)

Editor's Note: After graduating from nursing school in 1973, Patricia Kathleen (P.K.) Scheerle, RN, practiced pediatric intensive care nursing for the next seven years.

In 1980, P.K. left Vermont, and, on her way to California, stopped for two days in New Orleans. She's still there. In 1982 she founded American Nursing Services, Inc. (ANS), a supplemental staffing agency. ANS now has five offices in two states. P.K. has built ANS into a virtual empire, with services and future plans that are having a profound influence on the nursing profession and healthcare delivery nationwide.

NEE: Tell us about the events that led to your founding of ANS.
P.K.: "I came to New Orleans for two days on my way to California, and met someone with a company called Staff Builders. I started working for them, and on my second day, they asked if I would become their Director of Nursing. I thought this could be the wave of the future, so I worked for them for six months. By that time, I discovered that their way of running the business was not my way, so I went back to working PICU through another supplemental staffing agency called Allied Health.

After my first weekend, the company owner called and said, 'You did a phenomenal job at Staff Builders, would you run my company?' I jumped right on it—back then $30,000 a year was a mint. We went from being a large company without good details, to a very large business with good details and a lot of community respect. However, the company was sold eight months later. I was offered an administrative position, but, after meeting with the owners, I was not impressed enough to stay.

The CPA that negotiated that buy out approached me and said, 'If I co-sign a loan note with you, will you start your own company?' I said, 'Don't be silly, I'm a nurse.' And he said, 'I've watched you at both companies; at Allied Health you doubled revenues, and at Staff Builders you built it. You can do this, and nursing needs to govern itself.' I said, 'Well, that sounds like a fine idea; let's do it!'

We incorporated American Nursing Services in February, 1982. We started out providing supplemental staffing to ICU's. Then we opened an Educational Division that summer which taught ACLS and CCRN Review. We provided classes, not only to our own staff, but also free to our client's staff. We still do thirty classes a year. In August, we opened the Home Care Division and became Medicare/Medicaid certified. So, as you see, in 1982 we were building a one-stop shop.

In our first year of operation, our projected revenues were $400,000, and we did $1.3 million. We have doubled our size almost every year. We did $4.8 million in 1987, and this year we'll probably do $11.1 million."

NEE: To what do you attribute that kind of growth?
P.K.: "Eighty hours a week." [Laughs]

NEE: Your prior business experience must have helped.
P.K.: "I really didn't have any. I had no business responsibilities with those two companies; I was purely a director of nursing in clini-

cal areas. The reason I own ANS is because, out of seven founding nurses, no one was willing to co-sign the note except me. You see, I had no money—I came with everything I owned in a two-seater Fiat. I didn't know what $100,000 was all about so I signed the note and didn't worry. I was single, had no responsibilities, and figured what could they take? The bank said, 'What if your company dosen't make it?' and I said, 'I could pay you $100 a week for the rest of my life.' And, with a big co-signer, they went for it.

In February of 1983, on our first anniversary, my partner got married, wanted to make some changes, and came to me saying he wanted out. He must have notified the bank, because they called my note. I had forty-eight hours to raise $160,000. So I went to nine banks in my only blue suit. Eight banks laughed, and one said that I was relatively pretty and obviously intelligent, and could certainly find someone rich to marry so I wouldn't have all these worries."

NEE: So the banks wouldn't help. What did you do?
P.K.: "I thought, 'who do I know that's rich?' I remembered this surgeon who always liked me, so I called and asked if he would be my partner. He told me if Price-Waterhouse looked at my books and approved it, he would agree. I said, 'I've got forty-eight hours, so don't drag your feet.' He called later and said, 'Price-Waterhouse says it's the best deal I could make—I want 51 percent.' I said no. I told him it's my blood, my sweat, my everything—I take 50 percent, you take 50 percent. He said okay, and became a silent partner until we became rich in late 1984.

Then he came to me and said, 'I'm the doctor and you're the nurse, and you are going to stop always doing things your way.' Whoa! We agreed to a stock buy out plan, and if I couldn't come up with the money, he would buy out my stock. The first bank I went to gave me the money. So, I bought him out in February, 1985, and thus we became a wholly nurse-owned company."

NEE: What business savvy have you since learned that has contributed to your success?
P.K.: "Good intuitive skills—such as anticipating the market, anticipating the growth in the elderly population, anticipating the growth in ICU beds, and believing that people will rise to be what you expect of them."

NEE: Namely your nurses?
P.K.: "Namely my nurses. We took nurses who were frustrated, leaving the profession, and invited them to an elegant free dinner so they could just talk with other nurses. As you can imagine, our staff grew like mad.

What we do is empower people to make it their own. For example, when we set up home care I didn't say, 'Hey, I'm great, so I am going to run home care.' We empowered someone else and told them: you've got the financial backing, build it yourself.

We have three criteria for each of our RN's; one is that we always dress for image. Image was important since the day we began. The second thing is that we never make a commitment we can't keep. And sometimes, when you are looking at $50,000, that's tough to do. The third thing we did was to only hire people we would want to take care of our parents.

Another thing—those people we interviewed and didn't hire, we offered to help. They could buddy—free of charge—with one of our senior critical care people to get their skills back in line. We also aligned ourselves with quite a few male nurses who were having trouble getting the autonomy they wanted in the areas they were working. We became very successful as many males grew into administration in the early 1980s. They had been our nurses, and they had been given a chance.

We also try to divvy up the wacky stuff to everybody. For example, we got a call from a Japanese ship line that needed thirty cholera injections in the middle of the Gulf of Mexico, so we got a chopper and sent out a nurse. And the Republican National Convention called and said, 'We need you to be our nurses.' So we took our hardest workers and gave them that honor.

We also have a mechanism in our company for information referral. For instance, people will call us thinking we are the American Nurses Association and say, 'My daughter wants to be a nurse, what do I do?' Louisiana recently had a third-party reimbursement bill that failed, but we had a phone number we advertised that you could call for information. The same with the RCT problem now; you can call us and see what's going on."

NEE: What other areas have you delved into?
P.K.: "In October, 1987, we opened American Nursing Recruitment and Placement, which is in a separate office, but also based in New Orleans . It does nothing but place staff and executive nurses all over the country. We also place physical therapists and occupational therapists, and last week we got our first request for a hospital Chief Financial Officer. We opened our Dallas office in March of 1988, and in May we opened our respiratory therapists in all our client hospitals."

NEE: Are you contracting individual respiratory therapists, or staffing entire departments?
P.K.: "We're doing both."

NEE: Have you contracted nursing services to staff an entire unit yet?
P.K.: "Yesterday we got our first request to staff an eighteen-bed Recovery Room! So I will pull 100 recovery room nurses into my office, hand them a blank schedule, and say, 'This takes twenty-five full time equiva-

lents and a one year commitment—who wants it?'"

NEE: Incredible! What about the future?
P.K.: "The next thing will probably be rural nursing centers. We can put in a staff of approximately sixteen clinical nurse specialists. Each day the clinic would house different staff. And, on a capitated rate per year for an individual or a family, they could come and see those nurses anytime. Or, we could do it on a fee-for-service basis; that is still up in the air. So, if you're hypertensive, you can be managed at home."

NEE: Are you developing a Center model yet?
P.K.: "Yes. It's going to be great! The Cajun people love nurses, so we have a perfect pilot spot. The other thing on the horizon we're looking at, is to open in fifty cities simultaneously a one-stop service enabling elders to live at home. The service will provide a nurse, put bars in your bathroom, install heating/air-conditioning, wallpaper your house, everything So, if your elder living in Tampa is injured, and you live in California, you can have the next best thing to being there."

NEE: You are indeed making great strides for our profession.
P.K.: "Some powerful people don't think so, simply because I provide supplemental staffing. But what is the alternative?

I am successful at keeping dissident nurses happy—and in nursing. That is my greatest pride. I have nurses that tell the younger people, 'Don't leave nursing, try home care,' or 'Don't leave, try collaborative practice with physicians,' or 'Don't leave, this head nurse is really innovative.' It's so refreshing."

American Nursing Services, Inc.
3900 N. Causeway Blvd., Suite 650
Metairie, LA 70002
(504) 833-3100

234

Chapter 35

What Are You Going to Do With Your Life?

by Marion B. Dolan, RN

The mid-1950s were a time for me to decide what I wanted to be in life. My choice was obvious; I wanted to be a physician. It had been a dream during my teen years, and now my dad was asking, "What are you going to do with your life, Marion?"

My first reply: "I'm going to be a physician." "Oh no you're not," was his answer. "Why not?" I asked. "Because, you are a girl, and you'll get married, and then all that education will go to waste. Your brother will be the doctor in the family," Dad said. From tear-stained eyes I asked, "What will I do then?" He said, "You can be a nurse or a teacher. The choice is yours."

Some choices, I thought. For a few weeks I was entertaining thoughts of becoming a teacher. It was mainly because of all those holidays and summers off. Plus, the pile of presents from appreciative students loomed big on my list.

After checking out the classroom, it was determined by yours truly that nursing was much closer to the world I wanted to be in on a day-to-day basis. (I'd like to add here that my brother never did become a physician. Rather, he became a butcher...oh so Freudian! However, I do have a cousin who is a surgeon. We call him "slash and stitch.")

The year was 1960, and I began my nursing career at St. Mary's Hospital in New York City. After three years of study, the last thing I ever thought of becoming was a nurse entrepreneur. Come to think of it, I didn't even know what the word meant. My nursing career ran parallel to Cherry Ames. Emergency Room, Labor and Delivery, Pediatrics, ICU, Orthopedics, Medical Surgical, Rehabilitation and Psych were my habitats. I liked them all. To me, nursing was fun. It offered a chance to impact on others' lives in a positive fashion, and I threw myself into it with relish.

After twenty years of institutional nursing, I recognized that the only place my patients wanted to be was *home*. I took a dramatic career switch and moved into home health as the executive director of a small visiting nurse agency. It was a wonderfully exciting time in my life. There was so much to do for patients and families in community health. My new ideas were, however, hampered by a very conservative board. Lack of nursing understanding caused them to veto the new ideas of hospice, high tech, and shared housing.

Around the same time, the government passed the Omnibus Reconciliation Act, which opened the Medicare certification door to nurse entrepreneurs. As soon as this happened, I knew what I must do. Gathering together two excellent partners and financial backing, I opened Heritage Home Health in central New Hampshire. In September of 1982, we became a Medicare-certified home health agency.

Our start-up was difficult and adventurous. Problem areas were banks, insurance, and acquiring a medical director.

When we first went to the bank, we were told to go into arts and crafts and open a little cottage industry. We would have failed miserably at this since none of us had any talent along those lines. It took us trips to five banks before we were able to obtain financing.

Getting insurance was also difficult since many of the insurance company owners were on the local VNA Boards and resented any "turf" competition. To finally obtain insurance we had to go to a company more than 100 miles away. The same held true for an accountant. We ended up using accounting services in Connecticut. This was a lucky move for us, since we were able to engage the services of a firm very bright in healthcare financing matters.

To get a medical director, we had to ask more than ten physicians before one said yes. This all was very interesting as we had to market nurses in business as a legitimate entity. We finally ended up with an excellent physician who is still with us today.

We began initially by offering all services allowable under Medicare: Nursing, P.T., O.T., S.T., M.S.W., and home health aides. In addition, we offered hospice and a shared housing service called People Match. High tech was added as the field evolved. We started with four employees, and now, ten years later, employ more than fifty people.

The Health Care Financing Administration held a meeting of all new Region I home health agencies to orient us. We were so excited to meet the others who were opening new agencies. It was our expectation that these people would be all nurses taking the opportunity to chart their own course. Inside, the meeting held the giants of private duty care who were now seeking Medicare certification: Medical Personnel Pool, Upjohn, Superior Care, and yes, Heritage Home Health. It was exciting and frightening to know that we had come this far.

We began in a quaint, old Victorian home and last September moved to new, huge condominium offices in Meredith, New Hampshire.

We were successful because we never lost sight of our goal—*excellent patient care.* We are always willing to go the extra mile for the people who request our services. If it can be done at home, we'll do it! Word-of-mouth has been our referral strength. The discharge planners at the hospitals soon recognized the high quality of our care. We judge our agency by great patient outcomes.

As an administrator, I am always willing to take any risks necessary for the success of Heritage. Some success tips include: an excellent financial plan, hiring the right people, a marketing plan, excellent patient care, excellent healthcare accounting, community rapport, excellent legal services, and P-squared management (pats and praises).

Owning my business has given me the opportunity to get involved in the higher social circle of healthcare. As a nursing author (another talent I learned to cultivate and use effectively), I serve on the Advisory Board of *Nursing '91* magazine. Additionally, I serve on several state and federal boards. All of these activities and appointments enhance my agency.

International speaking is another side effect of owning Heritage, as I can speak out on issues and pursue goals unattainable before. My fields of expertise include Ethics, Pain, and Laughter. On an annual basis I speak to more than fifty different groups. Again, this adds to the visibility of my home health agency.

Last year we diversified into forming an Institute for Pain, Suffering, and Grief Research. We also have established a Painline with a state-wide toll-free number to offer assistance. Because 70 percent of patients enter the system for the relief of pain, it is crucial for a hospice/home health agency to relieve pain in the community. This branching out would not have been as simple if I didn't own the agency.

As I've ventured along the entrepreneurial path, I've found fun, excitement, and a happiness I never dreamed possible. I am still able to be the best nurse I can be. However, I have much more control over the practice outcomes of my nursing career than when I worked in an institution. I can be creative and innovative. My own business allows me to develop new products, programs, and processes which benefit patient care.

A nursing dream came true—starting my own home health agency. My future dream is to buy a hospital and make it not a medical center, but a *nursing* center. As a career nurse, I have seen my role develop in collaboration with the physician. I have seen that, as a nurse, I make a huge difference in people's lives. As for my dad, he took all this success in stride and was an ardent Heritage Home Health supporter until his death.

I think I knew I had arrived the day he said, "Marion, I'm so proud of you and the wonderful things you can do for your fellow man."

UPDATE 1997

We are now into our fifteenth year of operation! The continuing struggle of being a woman in business in health care is challenging but very rewarding. As our Medicare certified home health agency has grown so have additional entrepreneurial endeavors.

Two new corporations have been added: a private duty, non Medicare company in 1989 and a Medicare Certified Hospice in 1994. The adventure and knowledge gained in dealing with patients and families have its own benefits. In addition, I have staff that have shared their day to day lives with me, through engagements, weddings, births, deaths, divorce and graduations. We continue to support each other and look forward to another fifteen years.

Heritage Home Health
Meredith Square, Route 3, RFD 2, Box 540-7
Meredith, NH 03253-9603
(603) 279-4700

Chapter 36

Hemodialysis Company
Rises to the Top

(This profile appeared in the September 1989 issue of the *Nurse-Entrepreneur's Exchange*.)

Editor's Note: Karol Stein, RN, founded the acute hemodialysis service, Haemo-Stat, Inc., with $250 in 1976. Today, with offices in Los Angeles and New York, Haemo-Stat is the country's largest privately-owned acute hemodialysis service, and provides both primary and backup high quality care to over forty contracting hospitals.

NEE: The idea for Haemo-Stat came in 1976 when you received a call from a physician who had a patient needing dialysis and couldn't be transferred.
Karol: "Yes. The patient was very ill, on a ventilator, and they didn't want to transfer him. The physician thought that if I could come over, and we could somehow arrange for equipment, that he could just dialyze him there. So, I borrowed a machine from a manufacturer, borrowed some supplies, and we did it.

At first, I leased a machine and started out with a part-time secretary and another nurse to take call. It wasn't until I got a second machine that a light bulb went on, and I realized that I could make money."

NEE: How did you market yourself early on?
Karol: "Two ways. One was that the sales reps who sold dialysis

machines were helping me. When they sold a machine to a hospital, they would recommend me as the nurse to run it for them. So, I got some business where I supplied just the labor and worked as an independent contractor.

I also went out and peddled myself; I did cold calls and made lots of phone calls. For the first two years, I also worked full-time as a head nurse in a hospital hemodialysis unit until I got so busy that it became unmanageable.

One important point is that early on, I was debt free. I didn't need to borrow any money since I had a full-time job and ran the business out of my home. I see many people who start a business and go heavily into debt. For some businesses that's appropriate, but for me, it's a large part of why I didn't fail. And I had plenty of opportunities to fail, since in the beginning we would go weeks without clients."

NEE: You are successful because Haemo-Stat services are cost-effective. How do you save hospitals money?
Karol: "They avoid capital expenditures; they don't have to buy any equipment, they don't need to maintain an inventory, and they don't have to hire, train and retain a nurse to perform dialysis which is probably done on an episodic basis. Dialysis nurses are certified, like to specialize, and don't like to go work in Labor & Delivery when there is no dialysis to be done. So, most hospitals can't keep a staff if their dialysis is infrequent, which is usually the case. In larger hospitals, where they have their own staff, we provide backup for them.

If hospitals have their own staff and equipment, they are paying out tremendous amounts on on-call pay. Some hospitals are paying $100,000 a year in call pay just for nurses to sit around and wait. With us, they can eliminate call pay. We might cost a little more per treatment, but they have no other costs involved. We can also supply only the RN to dialyze a patient with the hospital's equipment, so that makes it very reasonable for a larger hospital to use us on that basis."

NEE: Are you still doing all your own marketing?
Karol: "Yes. I did have a full-time sales rep a couple of years ago, and it didn't work. He was not a nurse; he was a professional sales rep and couldn't do as good a job as I could. I think that in my kind of business you have to market yourself. Most of my business is done by referral, and the dialysis community is small. I am well known, they know I'm in charge, and I'm the person they need to talk to, so they don't want to talk to anyone else."

NEE: A major political issue you've had to face?
Karol: "The dialysis community had the notion that a nurse couldn't do this —that a company like mine had to be owned by a physician, or be corporately owned with physician medical directorship. I still confront that occasionally; someone will say, 'Who's your medical director?' and I say to them, "Dialysis is a nursing procedure, nurses know nursing best, nurses can manage themselves, and we don't need medical directorship to perform and practice nursing.'"

NEE: What is the future direction of hospital nursing and nurses in business?
Karol: "Nursing corporations. I've had a centrally owned nursing corporation for four years. Haemo-Stat has its own nursing shortage problem, and I see a decentralized nursing corporation as the answer to that shortage. I can bring in good, loyal people who have been with me for a long time, and we can own the business cooperatively.

In the hospital: in ICU, CCU, or the ER—I don't see any department it wouldn't work in. Dialysis clinics that are corporately owned that are satellite units are absolutely amazing places for it to happen, because they don't have all the hospital bureaucracy on top of them, and they're completely dependent on their nursing staff. I was telling someone in a dialysis unit about this, and they said, 'What a great idea! I'd never have to worry about the personnel department, payroll taxes, or benefits.'

When I started Haemo-Stat, I was a business corporation, because that was before nursing corporations were available. But when I opened the New York office, I *had* to be a nursing corporation—no one is allowed to be in any kind of business providing healthcare in New York unless you a medical or nursing corporation. The idea is to keep business people out of healthcare; they only want practitioners actually practicing nursing or medicine. It keeps a lot of the riffraff out."

NEE: Do you plan to open more offices?
Karol: "No. Because for the success of the New York office, the tremendous amount of work and travel required—and the fact I have children—I'm making a lifestyle choice not to do that. I've decided that I'm successful enough."

UPDATE 1997

I'm fine, still here, doing okay with challenges of managed care. We have 45 employees, one office, and pull in 2.5 million dollars annually.

I made a life-style choice to stay the same size with limited growth. So I closed my New York office. Now I offer peritoneal dialysis and apheresis services on the same basis as all businesses. I'm sorry that 209 and affirmative action hit the dust in my state (women-owned business helped me).

I would love to mentor, but have never been asked. Aside from that, I network very little now; instead I cocoon with my family, which now that I am established is my main concern, along with company survival and employees well-being.

Haemo-Stat, Inc.
13939 Victory Blvd.
Van Nuys, CA 91401
(818) 376-4033

Chapter 37

A Good Sign

by Karen L. Wetther, BSN, RN.

At the open house to celebrate the opening of my office in December of 1989, several friends commented admiringly that it must be wonderful to finally see my dream become a reality.

Oddly enough, however, I have to admit that I had never dreamed of having my own business, and I certainly never wanted to take on what I perceived as the complex and heavy responsibility associated with having an office and employees. What did I know about negotiating a lease, Worker's Compensation insurance, witholding taxes, hiring—and perhaps even firing—employees?

To explain how I made the transition from staff nurse to a legal nurse consultant who also lectures nationwide, I need to backtrack several years. Many people and events in my life have been instrumental in helping me to get to this point, essentially reaching goals I had never even imagined. I would venture to say that most, if not all, successful people are where they are not only because of their hard work, persistence, and willingness to make sacrifices and delay gratification, but also because of the help and encouragement of others who have crossed their path along the way.

I feel extremely fortunate to have been born into a loving and supportive family. My parents, who are my greatest fans and supporters, instilled in me as a child a positive spirit, good values, an interest in helping others, a strong work ethic, and a strong faith in God—all of which have helped to shape my business.

Just a few months after graduating with my BSN from Biola College in Southern California in 1971, I was diagnosed as having rheumatoid arthritis. I had just accepted my first position as an RN at the University of Illinois Medical Center in Chicago, and while many people would have been devastated at this news, I was actually relieved as I strongly suspected I had the disease, but could not convince any doctor to investigate it. That was a difficult year physically as I adjusted to my disease and medications and had the first of what would be several surgeries over the next decade.

It was fortunate that the disease had an insidious onset, as this allowed me to continue with a nursing career over the next nine years. Without that clinical experience which included pediatrics, med/surg, orthopedics, discharge planning, newborn nursery, and a year of school nursing in Taichung, Taiwan, I would not have been equipped to work as a legal nurse consultant.

My arthritis continued to progress, making hospital nursing increasingly difficult. My co-workers often had to make special allowances for me as I could not lift as much as was often necessary, so I sometimes required a lighter assignment. The long and often cruel Chicago winters were also difficult, so I began to make plans to move to San Diego, California, in 1978. I had spent most of my childhood and adolescent years on the tropical island of Guam, and I was anxious to return to a warm climate with ocean and palm trees. However, my plans were disrupted when several of my MCP joints were dislocated. I remained in Chicago for another year to undergo joint replacement surgeries in both hands.

In May, 1979, I was finally ready to relocate, and drove cross-country to San Diego. I knew only one person there, but had also convinced my sister to move there, and I quickly made new friends when

I took a position in the Newborn Nursery on the night shift at UCSD Medical Center. I thoroughly enjoyed that unit and my co-workers, who again were kind enough to make allowances for me. It was there that I became friends with an RN who, eight years later, became my assistant when I started my business and has assisted me at every workshop since April of 1987.

In July of 1980, I took what was supposed to have been a five-week leave of absence to have more hand surgery, as two of the joint replacements had already fractured. Due to complications, I was unable to return to work as soon as expected. One Saturday night in November, my supervisor called me at home to kindly forewarn me that I would be receiving a letter informing me that the hospital would no longer be able to hold my position and would have to terminate me for medical reasons. I recall feelings of shock, panic, and anger as I looked ahead to an unknown future. To add insult to injury, a clerical error at the hospital resulted in the cancellation of my health insurance rather than conversion to an individual policy. No job, no health insurance, a pre-existing condition with the possibility of further surgery— this was one of the lowest points in my life.

I was on Social Security disability, attempting to live on my $700 monthly check supplemented by my savings. Over the next two years I underwent three more hand surgeries, each of which was followed by approximately three months of intensive occupational therapy.

While I was recovering from one of my surgeries in the spring of 1982, a friend visited me in the hospital. When she returned home that afternoon she mentioned to her husband, a personal injury attorney, that she wondered whether I would ever be able to work in the hospital again. He said that his law firm had been thinking about hiring a nurse to summarize medical records for them, so she called me while I was still in the hospital and asked if I might be interested in doing that. I thanked her for thinking of me and promised to think about it, but, in all honesty, I could not get very excited about the thought of helping attorneys—and I was afraid that I would really miss having patient contact. The prospect of sitting in a room all day poring over medical records sounded absolutely boring! However, I knew I would have to find some type of work, and this would at least allow me to use my medical knowledge, so I decided to look into it.

In January, 1983, three months after my final surgery, I interviewed with two of the attorneys in the nine-attorney firm. Armed with the resume I had so carefully prepared and a copy of my nursing license, neither of which they were even remotely interested in, we talked for a few minutes, and they hired me on the spot. (I should mention here that things have changed since then, and most attorneys do want to see professional-looking resumes of prospective legal nurse consultants.)

On January 7, 1983, I began my career as a legal nurse consultant at the law offices of Wingert, Grebing, Anello and Chapin in downtown San Diego, a position that unbeknownst to me at the time, was to dramatically change my life. I later found that I was the first RN in San Diego to work full-time for a law firm, and I did not meet another legal nurse consultant until more than three years later, when we found ourselves on opposite sides of a very intense case which went to trial.

When I initially took the position with the law firm, I was given about twenty minutes of on-the-job training by one of the attorneys, and from that point on I learned by trial and error and by soliciting feedback from the attorneys. I had no legal background and, while this did not concern the two attorneys who hired me, it was a concern to the other attorneys in the firm—consequently, they would not allow me to work on their cases at the outset. However, it was not long before they started giving me cases also.

I loved the job, to my surprise, and actually felt I had found my niche. Where being thorough and detail-oriented had sometimes been a detriment in the acute-care setting, I was elated to have found a career alternative in which I could use my nursing knowledge and experience, and in which I could capitalize on my strengths.

Nurses began asking me how I had gotten into such an interesting career, what I actually did for the attorneys, and how they might enter the field. Several took me to lunch to "pick my brain" and I began spending more time than I could really allow to share the information. I believe it was my mother who suggested that perhaps I should consider giving workshops to groups of nurses as a solution to the problem.

The idea appealed to me because I've always enjoyed teaching, but I knew nothing about starting a business. I wanted to do everything right, so I enrolled in two courses over the next few months. One was offered at a local hospital and was entitled "Effective Presentation Skills" and the other was an eight-week Small Business Management certificate program offered by a local university. Using some of the suggestions from the first course, I developed a one-day workshop for nurses on Medical Legal Consulting.

I officially started my home-based business, which I called Medical Legal Resources, in February on 1987. I wanted to have the word *resources* in my business name because, according to Webster, it means "a source of help and supply," and this is how I hoped it would be viewed by nurses and attorneys alike. It was financed with approximately $2,000, a portion of a settlement from an auto accident. While the accident was a terrible inconvenience at the time and for several months thereafter, I now see it as a blessing in disguise because it provided the finances to start my modest business at just the right time. I used the money to hire a graphic artist to design a logo, purchase business cards and stationery, file a fictitious name statement and obtain a business license, pay the application fee to the California Board of Registered Nursing so that I could offer continuing education credits, rent a mailbox, establish myself with a reputable and professional answering service, and for various courses and other necessary supplies.

The first year I conducted four workshops in San Diego. In 1988, when a California nursing publication published an article about medical legal nurse consulting which included information from an interview with me, I started receiving calls from nurses throughout the state asking when I would be offering a workshop in their area. I made the decision to branch out slowly and offered one in Northern California and one in Orange County, both of which were well attended. In 1989 I offered one in Chicago—my first out-of-state workshop—and, as a result of an article I had written for an Illinois nursing publication, there was so much interest that we returned to do another workshop there two months later.

It was during 1989 that I began feeling overwhelmed trying to work at the law firm and keep up with my own business. I attended the National Nurses in Business Association conference in San Francisco in March and was amazed and energized by the nurse entrepreneurs who had already done so much and were terrific role models for those of us who were new to enterpreneurship. The following month I was a speaker at a conference co-sponsored by the Emory University School of Nursing and the Nurses in Business Association in Atlanta. Again I was stimulated and encouraged to see what nurse entrepreneurs were doing and how they were doing it. While I was still hesitant to take on the responsibility of an office and employees, the thought did cross my mind that I could probably handle one or two employees after seeing how other nurses had started businesses which employed hundreds of people.

When I returned from Atlanta, I contacted a business consultant who had been one of my instructors in the Small Business Management certificate program and met with her soon after to discuss some ideas and obtain assistance in expanding my business. We developed a business plan, and it became clear to me that I would need to lease office space. If I had only a consulting practice I could have continued to work out of my home, but the expanding workshop facet of the business would require more space and at least one employee.

One of the nice things about working with business consultants is that they will do a lot of the groundwork. They looked for office space, took my figures, and developed a proforma showing the best and worst case scenarios financially, obtained information on phone services available for my type of practice, etc. I just did not have time to do this myself since I was juggling the law firm position and my business and was already working twelve to fourteen hours per day during the week, and an average of four to six hours a day on weekends.

Many people who did not have businesses were unable to understand why I would work so hard. Unless one has had the experience to create something from nothing and watch it grow, it is difficult to understand, but while it was exhausting, I also found it exhilarating! By that time I was talking to nurses from all over the country on a daily basis. I thoroughly enjoyed that, and still do.

We were finally ready to try to secure a business loan from the bank. One of the services offered gratis by my business consultant is arranging and attending the appointment with a banker. She selected a bank which she felt might be open to at least offering a line of credit to a relatively new business owner. Unfortunately, the banker wasn't willing to take the risk, although he assured me that he thought I would be successful. I was so devastated that I wanted to give up the whole idea.

I was in the process of convincing myself that I was crazy to think that any bank would be willing to give me a loan since I had essentially no assets, having depleted my savings during my period of disability and subsequently putting all my money into the business. However, my consultant was confident that we could do it, and promptly set up an appointment with another banker. She again went with me, and that banker agreed to look over my business plan and notify me of his decision the following week. The waiting was very difficult, but he called five days later and said he had decided to approve a line of credit for $15,000.

When I went in to sign the papers, he told me that I did not fit any of their criteria and he would not ordinarily have approved my loan. However, the three things which convinced him to take a risk were that I had excellent credit, I had excellent credentials for this type of business, and I was very employable, so if my business did fail I could get a job and repay the loan with my wages. I was ecstatic, grateful, and motivated to prove to him that he had made the right decision.

After signing the loan papers, I went to the office I was planning to lease and signed those papers. What an exciting day September 7, 1989, was for me! The next day I submitted my resignation to the law firm and officially opened my office for business on October 2, 1989.

Since then the business has continued to grow. I began repaying my loan after six months and was able to hire a full-time receptionist/secretary after fourteen months. Prior to that, my mother had held that position on a part-time basis, helping me through those early months. In addition to offering workshops across the country each month, I continue to assist attorneys and forensic physicians with the medical aspects of their cases. I am also asked to speak at conferences and to the nursing staff at various hospitals on an increasingly frequent basis.

I have learned a lot since the inception of my business, and would offer the following recommendations to prospective entrepreneurs:

> * Be willing to invest time and money to learn from reputable consultants and take courses before and after starting your business to learn all you can.

      * Do not expect to make large profits for quite some time. Do expect to work long hours. If you have a passion for your venture, you will probably do it willingly.

      * Listen to the advice of others, but follow your own intuition.

      * Listen to your clients and prospective clients and try to anticipate and meet their needs.

      * Be willing to share. What you give to others will come back to you many times over. As an entrepreneur, I've laughed, I've cried, I've bitten my nails waiting for the money to come in—but I have never once asked myself why in the world I went into business for myself. I think that's a good sign!

UPDATE 1997

The intervening years since I wrote "A Good Sign" have offered me a kaleidoscope of experiences, emotions and opportunities which have resulted in both personal and professional growth. Some of the experiences were wonderful. Others were so difficult that I would not choose to repeat them in my lifetime, yet I have to admit that they have taught me a lot, increased my inner strength and will help me to relate to others who find themselves in circumstances similar to those I found myself in.

1997 is the year of my 10th year anniversary in business, so writing this epilogue now is very timely. So many opportunities which relate to the field of legal nurse consulting have presented themselves over the last two years that I now have the luxury of choosing those which I enjoy the most. (I think it's the nurse in me that wants to try to tackle them all!)

I prefer to focus on the positive in life. Because this book is meant to help aspiring and established nurse entrepreneurs, however, I would be remiss if I excluded some of the challenges I have faced over the past five years while sharing only the positive experiences and opportunities.

At the end of 1990, I was operating under the misconception that I was home free since my small business had remained viable for four years. That is what many banks and other business professionals often lead you to believe. That of course, did not take into account the possibility of an unexpected lengthy illness, a potentially devastating economic recession or a personal crisis, all of which I experienced between 1991 and 1994. It is now my belief that one should never assume their business is home free, since unexpected things can and probably will occur which may adversely affect ones business.

The series of challenges I faced started in January of 1991 when my body protested the fact that I was working an average of twelve to sixteen hours per day (not unusual for an entrepreneur). I had a major flare of my rheumatoid arthritis which decreased my productivity to three to five hours per day. On the heels of that illness came the recession, which adversely affected my business in 1992 and 1993. My two markets (attorneys and nurses) dropped, as everyone seemed to be holding on tightly to their money, and my best client, from whom I received about 1/3 of my cases and income, was forced to give up his practice. Many well-meaning friends suggested that I go back to work for someone else, but I was determined to ride out the storm. I read a book entitled *How To Survive the Recession* shortly after I started feeling the effects of the recession and adopted the author's belief that 90% of surviving it was the belief and determination to do so.

The economy started improving very gradually toward the end of 1993 and I was sure that the worst was over and was very anxiously anticipating a great year in 1994! In January of 1994, however, a very dear friend who has had a major impact on my life died of a serious illness at the age of 43 and I learned that another friend had contracted AIDS secondary to a violent sexual assault. I was devastated and I was physically and emotionally exhausted by this time. However, with the support of God, my loving and supportive family, my rheumatologist, friends and colleaugues, I carried on and eventually things did take a turn for the better—MUCH better.

Somehow in 1994 I wrote a 260-page "how-to" manual, *The Nuts & Bolts of Legal Nurse Consulting,* and worked with an advisory board of legal nurse consultants and nurse attorneys to develop and coordinate the first Legal Nurse Consultant Certificate Program in the country, offered by the University of California at San Diego Extension. Both have been very successful and are very satisfying for me. In 1996 I contributed two chapters to the book which will serve as the core curriculum for the American Association of Legal Nurse Consultants' certification program. I continue to consult with attorneys on the medical aspects of their cases, give a few training workshops each year, speak at conferences, and I love receiving calls from nurses all over the country and in Canada who need a little mentoring and encouragement as they take the plunge into this exciting nursing specialty. I'm even making an attempt at writing a novel in my spare time!

My very best advice to an aspiring entrepreneur would be to find something to do that you are absolutely passionate about and would almost be willing to do for no remuneration. You may have to at some point and the passion will help you through the really rough times.

Medical Legal Resources
6565 Riverdale Street
San Diego, CA 92120
(619) 584-6489

Chapter 38

A Spa Retreat

(This profile appeared in the May 1989 issue of the *Nurse-Entrepreneur's Exchange.*)

Editor's Note: Southwind Health Resort is a nationally-acclaimed women's spa established in 1986 by Doreen MacAdams, RN, MSN. Located just north of Atlanta, Georgia, the 1985 renovated eight-bedroom Victorian house sits on sixteen beautiful acres bordering Lake Allatoona. Ms. MacAdams was named 1989 Outstanding Young Working Woman by **Glamour Magazine.**

NEE: Why did you decide to start a health resort?
Doreen: "I had been involved in CCU and cardiac rehab, and after I became a nurse practitioner, I went into private practice with a group of cardiologists. I enjoyed the rehab, but felt I would have a greater impact doing preventative medicine, because no matter what you tell the man who's had a heart attack about diet or exercise, it would never get through unless you could get to the wife. So I started a women's spa to get to the whole family."

NEE: How did you decide on the Atlanta area for the resort's location?
Doreen: "I was living in New York, and decided to move south because the weather is better and the cost of living is lower. I decided on the Atlanta area because it was a wonderful market since there are no other spas here, the weather is nice, and the cost of property was low compared to the Northeast."

Nee: What did your marketing research consist of?
Doreen: "I visited many spas in New York, Florida, Connecticut, and others on the East Coast. I then developed our program by synthesizing the best aspects of those, along with my own ideas of what a resort should offer.

To run this kind of business, I had to get the property commercially zoned, since it was originally zoned residential. So I had to get the neighbors to sign a petition stating they weren't in opposition, and then present the proposal before the zoning board."

NEE: Did you run into much neighborhood opposition?
Doreen: "No, because we improved the property value of the area. What people really wanted to know was that a Holiday Inn wasn't going in next door. I also reassurred them that there wouldn't be any drinking or late night parties, so there wasn't any problem at all."

NEE: What's the essence of Southwind's program?
Doreen: "We deal with four different levels; the physical—with exercise and fitness—and the psychological/emotional through our seminars. Then we get into stress reduction and relaxation offering massage and beauty services. The fourth component of the program is sound nutrition. We offer balanced meals, and our nutritionist takes the women to the grocery store and teaches them how to shop properly.

The focus of the spa is educational, but the women are actually living the experience. We don't focus our *marketing* on the educational aspect, because that's not why people go to a spa. Most come because they are stressed out or overweight, or want to get re-motivated, or just get away from it all.

But to achieve this, and to change people for the rest of their lives, we get them into an ideal setting—we're out in the country, there's plenty of time to exercise, and we feed them low calorie gourmet meals. They have the time to take good care of themselves, and they feel wonderful while they are doing it. It's a very positive experience for change."

NEE: What topics do you cover in your seminars?
Doreen: "We cover stress reduction, emotional overeating, our dietician teaches how to eat out properly, and we have a cardiologist and a physical therapist teaching cardiovascular fitness. Then we have fun seminars, such as Wardrobe Accessorizing, Dressing for Your Body Type, the Psychology of Color, and even Astrology. We have two psychiatric nurse practitioners who cover goal setting, communication, and relationships. We try to present topics that are appropriate to all women."

NEE: How do you market Southwond?
Doreen: "Mostly through regional and national ads. Also, this month we're featured in *Cosmopolitan, Complete Woman, Shape,* and *American Health.* Next month we will be in *Savvy* and *Entrepreneur.*"

Nee: How did you accomplish such a marketing sweep?
Doreen: "The spring is the best season for getting back into shape, so this is the time magazines want to cover spas and health resorts. But many of the features are the result of years of writing press re leases, talking with people, and doing follow up. We've been trying for years to get into *Cosmopolitan,* and we just now made it."

Nee: What has been your biggest business challenge?
Doreen: "Employee relations! I was used to working with nurses, with whom you deal on a professional level. Lay people don't think or react the same way. Some don't want to think at all—they want you to be responsible and take the heat. When a crisis happens, and it is five o'clock, they just throw up their hands and beat it.
The point I'm making is that we deal with many different levels of employees, and in the hotel business the domestic stuff is always difficult. You are dealing with many different personalities, and you

have to learn how to get the best out of people. It can be very time consuming."

NEE: What does the future hold for Southwind?
Doreen: "Next year we want to build on an addition so that we can house more customers. Once that's done, we want to open another resort somewhere. We haven't decided on a specific site yet."

NEE: What makes Southwind unique?
Doreen: "Some spas just pamper you, with very little focus on exercise or nutrition. Others are into total fitness only. Our focus is wider; we try to appeal to women on all different levels. If you are not a fitness nut, you can go to the cooking classes, participate in the seminars, or just hang out on the porch. So, even though we have many different activities, people can participate in as few or many as they wish—it's their choice."

Chapter 39

A Roller Coaster Ride
Into Business

by Pamela M. Buckman, RN, MS

I would love to be able to say that I started my own business based on a well thought out plan for sucess, but it simply isn't true!

A Harvard MBA always sounded to me like a lab test for an exotic disease. During my twelve years of clinical nursing, I have never attended a business class, never raised capital, never written a business plan for my own company, and have never been able to fully grasp the nuances of an intricate financial statement without significant hand holding from my accountant. Even so, I have been in business for ten years and never known a month "in the red." In retrospect, I recognize that I have what it takes to start a business and make it successful.

The word that leaps to mind most readily to describe my entrance into business is *survival*. My nursing career was a predictable eighteen-month roller coaster ride through changes in specialties, areas of employment, positions, and responsibilities. I spent six months learning a new job, six months doing the job, and six months looking for the next challenge. I always loved what I was doing because it was constantly new. I made sure I didn't get bored. When ever the challenge and/or fun began to wane, I made a change, although starting a business did not occur to me during those years. I was merrily working away just like everyone else I knew. I married, had two children, and became the sterotypical, second-income wage earner. And then two things happened. I chose to place myself smack dab in the middle of one of the most prevalent of women's problems in America today. I became a single mother with two pre-school children and the primary (sole more often than not) breadwinner. I could no longer live with rotating shifts, weekend and holiday work with financial disaster as my reward. Even more importantly, I couldn't see it would ever be any different if I didn't make a significant career change, and so I did.

I am forever grateful to my mom, who saw an ad from a local medical device firm in the classified section of the Sunday paper. They were looking for a master's level nurse who was familiar with research, cardiovascular, and orthopaedic nursing. (Thank goodness for that extra two years in school and all those specialty changes during my roller coaster days.) I threw together a resume (never having done one before) and submitted it to the company. They sent me an application for employment, which I completed and hand delivered to a receptionist one morning. I was wearing jeans and tennis shoes, since I had little confidence this would actually lead to anything. Much to my surprise, two weeks later I hung up my white uniform for the last time and joined the business world.

My position involved the management of clinical trial programs to evaluate company products in satisfaction of Food and Drug Administration regulations. I was inundated with information—all of which was brand new to me. I not only had to learn my job, I had to learn to do my job in a foreign country, i.e., an office. As if traveling to a foreign country, I read, watched, and listened with a renewed interest in work that I had not realized was being done. I felt challenged and motivated to learn, produce and to do whatever was required to excel—whether or not the work could be done in forty hours a week.

I also learned to travel and juggle a home life at the same time. This is not an easy task for anyone, and indisputably impossible without a supportive family, which, luckily I had.

The occupational hazards of working for someone else in the business world soon came my way. Within two years, the company was sold and relocated. I went to work for another medical device firm doing essentially the same thing. That medical division was below the acceptable profit margin level for the board of directors of the parent company, and the division was dis

And then two things happened. I chose to place myself smack dab in the middle of one of the most prevalent of women's problems in America today. I became a single mother with two pre-school children and the primary (sole more often than not) breadwinner. I could no longer live with rotating shifts, weekend and holiday work with financial disaster as my reward. Even more importantly, I couldn't see it would ever be any different if I didn't make a significant career change, and so I did.

I am forever grateful to my mom, who saw an ad from a local medical device firm in the classified section of the Sunday paper. They were looking for a master's level nurse who was familiar with research, cardiovascular, and orthopaedic nursing. (Thank goodness for that extra two years in school and all those specialty changes during my roller coaster days.) I threw together a resume (never having done one before) and submitted it to the company. They sent me an application for employment, which I completed and hand delivered to a receptionist one morning. I was wearing jeans and tennis shoes, since I had little confidence this would actually lead to anything. Much to my surprise, two weeks later I hung up my white uniform for the last time and joined the business world.

My position involved the management of clinical trial programs to evaluate company products in satisfaction of Food and Drug Administration regulations. I was inundated with information—all of which was brand new to me. I not only had to learn my job, I had to learn to

265

do my job in a foreign country, i.e., an office. As if traveling to a foreign country, I read, watched, and listened with a renewed interest in work that I had not realized was being done. I felt challenged and motivated to learn, produce and to do whatever was required to excel—whether or not the work could be done in forty hours a week.

I also learned to travel and juggle a home life at the same time. This is not an easy task for anyone, and indisputably impossible without a supportive family, which, luckily I had.

The occupational hazards of working for someone else in the business world soon came my way. Within two years, the company was sold and relocated. I went to work for another medical device firm doing essentially the same thing. That medical division was below the acceptable profit margin level for the board of directors of the parent company, and the division was disad or conducted a direct-mail program. In a sense, we never directly marketed our services.

And so, there I was still working weekends and holidays. The difference was I now worked fourteen to sixteen hour days and six to seven days a week. But that was not the only difference. More importantly, I was no longer bored. I thoroughly enjoyed entering into a contract to do a job, completing that job with integrity, on time, within budget, and being handsomely rewarded for my efforts.

It is now ten years later. We have a staff of seven, a very nice, but not extravagant, fully equipped suite of offices, an extensively networked computer system, and multiple opportunities for further expansion.

Have we made mistakes along the way? You bet, and plenty of them! We sold a piece of the company to an accountant because we were naive to the telltale signs of manipulation. It cost us dearly to buy back that piece of the company. We hired the wife of a friend. The wife turned out to be incompetent. Firing the wife cost us the friendship. We loaned money to friends, never dreaming we would have to threaten legal action to be repaid.

But we obviously did more things right than wrong. We controlled our overhead with a vengeance and continue to do so. We put money into people—not furniture. We were patient. Our slow, constant growth was controllable and therefore predictable. We never hired an employee until we exhausted every possibility of doing the work ourselves. We watched and listened to other successful small business owners—and learned from them.

In the early days, I personally had many opportunities to meet with small groups of nurses who talked about wanting to start their own businesses. Some of them had taken the first steps to establish themselves. I remember being amazed at comments such as: "I won't travel over a weekend," or "I won't travel at all," or "My hours are 8-5," or "I won't work with someone I don't like."

These comments do not embody the entrepreneur spirit. In contrast to the above, my philosophy has always been: *Work wherever the work is and whenever the work needs to be done.* To borrow a saying from a successful friend of mine: "Where is it written that associates must always be friends? It is only necessary to do good business." This dosen't mean you should agree to work with unethical or otherwise undesirable individuals. It does mean that you must develop the proper perspectives. Business associates do not have to stand up to the same scrutiny as candidates to date your daughter. By the way, among those nurses I met who made the remarks I found so amazing, none have been successful in their own businesses. Owning your own business involves long, hard, endless hours of work and responsibility. Being willing to work that hard is not enough. You have to thrive on it. It has to be fun!

Would I do it again? You bet. Could I work for someone else again? Of course—I am a survivor—but I don't plan to have to make that choice.

267

If I were to use one word to capture the feeling that embodies being a entrepreneur, it is *caring*. The successful owner conceives, delivers, nurtures and develops the business like a lioness with her pride. She is protective and defensive. Success depends on delegation of authority and responsibility to others. But, in the end, no one benefits and no one fails any more or any less than the extent to which the entrepreneur *cares*.

UPDATE 1997

I wrote my story for the original publication of *50 Tales* while riding on an airplane between San Francisco and New York. It seemed only fitting that I write the follow-up to my story, once again at 30,000+ feet in the air—compliments of United Airlines. The truth is I spend at least 60% of my time in a pressurized cabin on my way to or from my friendly Marriott!

I have been in this "fast lane" for 20 years and I still love it. I have traveled to every state in the U. S. and to many other continents as well. My excess accumulation of frequent flyer points has provided free travel for my parents, in-laws, children and friends to take vacations that were otherwise out of consideration for them. The opportunity to do this for them is wonderful and makes me feel great!

Such things are clearly the benefits of business entrepreneurship and I take full advantage of them. At the same time, there is a price to pay . I continue to work long hard hours. I continue to accept risks—personal and financial. I continue to make hard decisions. Thank God, most of them are good. On the downside since my original writing, my company has been named in a class-action lawsuit. One of my lucrative clients cut corners and produced dangerous medical equipment, forcing us to drop the account for our own ethical reasons. Another lucrative client dropped us when their own research was poor and inconclusive; they needed someone to blame. What's the bottom line? There is no free lunch.

So—where does all this lead? Upward and onward, of course! Once you start down the entrepreneurial path, there is no turning back. I have seen it written that we all experience at least three separate careers in our lifetime. As I write this, I am motivated, excited, enthusiastic and delighted to say that I am headlong aimed at career #3.

My first career (and my core) was nursing (14 years). My second career was consulting on clinical research and FDA regulatory requirements for medical products (20 years). For my third career, I am now positioned to launch a product into the healthcare consumer market. The product is unique, simple, disposable, and inexpensive. I am immersed the idiosyncratic language of the venture capitalists, IPOs, consumer packaging, advertising agencies and multimedia promotions! It is all relatively new. It is a steep learning curve. And yes, I am (again!) going out on a financial limb.

What sets the entrepreneur apart is the fun and excitement that risk represents as opposed to the anxiety it provokes in the less adventuresome. Is there stress? Of course! But stress for the entrepreneur is motivating rather than disabling. Anyone considering an entrepreneurial life style must make some up-front decisions. If you want security, set hours, weekends off, guarantees and praise from others, you are better suited to be an employee. If the thrill of the chase is a goal unto itself, go for it! You may be an entrepreneur waiting to happen.

The Buckman Company, Inc.
1000 Burnett Avenue, Suite 250
Concord, CA 94520
(415) 372-7740

Chapter 40

A Strong Sense of Porpoise

by Sandra Ritz, RN, MS, MPH

I've always envied people who, from the moment they left the birth canal, knew what they wanted to be when they grew up. Maybe the fact that I was born on an elevator contributed to the ups and downs of my career choices.

As a child, I had good role models: my mom's an artist, my dad an accountant. About the only thing I could do well was paint by numbers. Maybe that influenced my drift into creative entrepreneurship. I sold handmade coloring books and toys to the neighborhhod kids. Circumstances fueled this endeavor; my sisters and I did not get an allowance. We had to learn to earn our spending money.

I charged parents a quarter per kid for costumes in plays I wrote and directed starring their children. I "borrowed" some of mom's clothes and pocketed the costume costs. My favorite production was "The little Engine That Could." I always played the clown, cheerleading the train to "think it can." Each play was a fun fiasco, and I made additional money from parent admission fees. My entrepreneur skills were not yet finely honed, though I didn't realize that during those many weeks of daily after-school rehearsals I could have charged babysitting time as well. Like early toilet training for nursing, it was already preparing me to not consider direct reimbursement payments for taking care of others.Fate and iatrogeny (medical-induced disease) influenced my decision to go into nursing. Always healthy as a child, I was devastated when diagnosed with cervical cancer on my twenty-first birthday. Repeated surgical procedures ensued, and the only humane treatment I remember having was from nurses. I fought to keep my uterus, hand carrying slides of slices of my cervix to different pathologists. I won the fight to keep my body intact; surgery had removed all the cancer. However, it was found that I had terotogenic deformity caused by a drug to prevent miscarriage (DES), which was prescribed to my mother while pregnant with me. It had caused the development of abnormal structures in my reproductive system and led to the cancer. I was branded in-utero by DES, condemned to a life-long dependence on medical care.

Public efforts nationally to obtain financial assistance for DES daughters' medical bills were fruitless. One attorney filed a suit for me and other DES daughters against several pharmaceutical companies. I could foresee how ugly it could get—my first deposition was with nine male attorneys, all asking me embarrasing and intimidating questions about my sexual habits. Once I knew that the cancer was gone and that my medical care expenses in the future would be within reason, I dropped the case. I had no desire to put my cervix up in court against a large drug company. I was glad to be alive and ready to go on with my life. I went back to school, taking pre-nursing courses. I figured becoming a nurse would give me some power as a patient as well as an opportunity to empower others in similar circumstances.

To earn money for nursing school, I leased a catering truck and sold lunches at the county hospital which had a lousy cafeteria. I made extra money selling homemade cookies. I was always told to "keep the change" when I told my nurse customers about my aspiring nursing career. Interestingly, the doctors never gave me any tips.

I guess I started dabbling in nurse entrepreneurship while still in nursing school. At that time I didn't know that I was being an entrepreneur, which, according to Funk and Wagnalls, is "one who undertakes to start and conduct an enterprise or business." I just knew that there were needs to be filled and bills to be paid.

On my first day of clinical training in the hospital, my instructor kicked me off the floor because I didn't have a name tag. I had no money, so I went home and made one. The next day there was a big pow-wow with nursing administration over my custom name tag. It had my name and proper title as required. But my instructor thought the hand-painted Peter Max scene between the lines was less than professional. As there was no specific rule in the books against pretty-pictured name tags, I got to wear it. By the end of my shift I had thirty-four orders. By my fourth clinical week, almost everyone in the hospital had ordered a custom name tag (including the director of nursing), and I had enough money for books, tuition, and rent for the rest of the year. Not only did I begin to comprehend the business concept of *find a need and fill it,* I recognize the possibilities of the marketing concept of *create a need to fill.*

My artistic side tired of the name tag business when I realized I couldn't keep making money unless I moved towards mass production. My entrepreneurial desires have always been closely tied to opportunities to exercise my creativity; I found it no longer challenging if they were all going to be the same. My delight as an artist was in creating something unique to the wearer. My name tag business moved down to hobby status as I set out to make a salary in the art of nursing.

An exploding bedpan hopper convinced me that staff nursing was not for me; I never could get all those stains out of my uniform. So, I entered an OB-GYN nurse practitioner program and was back to hungry student status again. My inherited artistic talent paid off—I painted signs for local restaurant windows in exchange for meals.

Burnout came within a year of my first nurse practitioner job. I just couldn't do another pelvic, especially since the physicians making the money wanted me to do those exams faster and more frequently (for the same salary). So much for the art of nursing.

With visions of Gauguin dancing in my head, I went to Tahiti. No more nursing; I was going to sell photographs and handpainted T-shirts. Within a week, I was dispensing Pepto-Bismol to fellow travelers and volunteering at the island infirmary. That nursing curse was in my blood—I could not ignore my skills in caring. I spent two years in Tahiti working as a volunteer nurse consultant for the French government, a nurse at Club Med, and an on-location nurse for a Hollywood film company.

Back to the U.S.A. and I knew I didn't want to work strictly in OB-GYN anymore. My interests were in self-care education, helping patients and their families regain control over their lives. So I went back to school in 1979, getting a master's in Public Health and master's degree in Nursing at the University of Hawaii. I got involved in media and health, including writing health articles and a stint as on-air nurse and researcher on Dr. Dean Edell's radio show. I learned the value of health advocacy through the mass media, educating people through radio and TV about toxic shock syndrome and tampon use.

Then I took a job for four years as a clinical nurse specialist working with chronic back pain patients. This was my most creative and rewarding nursing job. Everything in medicine had already been tried for these patients and failed, so I was given free reign. I found that if I could make them laugh—see the absurdity—they would get better. I was the clown again, telling them to "think I can." I helped them gain control over their pain, rather than their pain controlling them. I also intervened to coordinate their care between the many doctors, lawyers, and insurance company adjustors involved. My interventions succeeded in helping many of these chronic pain patients get out of doctors' offices and return to the mainstream of life.

This, unfortunately, led to another prescription for nursing burnout. Administration's response to my success was to increase my patient load, decrease the time I could spend with each one, and give me no help and no pay incentive to work harder and longer. The prescription was soon filled and refills added; my daily patient load was increased even more. I was feeling sad and fatigued. But this time I was older and wiser. I filed a worker's compensation claim for "job stress" and went to half-time. We negotiated a token settlement to drop the case altogether, and with that money I bought a computer and office equipment. My living room became the office of my new company, Back Care Hawaii. I gradually picked up work with physicians, consulting with their chronic pain patients, and once I knew I could make enough to pay the rent, I left the half-time job completely.

Although I enjoyed working as a consultant, I was still dependent on physicians for my income. I could not get direct reimbursement for my income. I could not get direct reimbursement for my nursing care to pain patients; the physician would pay me an hourly rate to see his patients, and then bill in his name at a much higher rate. Attorneys would send large sets of medical records to a physician for review; the physician would pay me $30 an hour to organize and summarize them. With my experience in back care, I would also write recommendations on care. The physician would then turn around and bill the attorney up to $150 an hour for my time. My expertise was making me a living and making others rich.

In 1985 I became involved with community theater, first as a volunteer stage manager for a fast-paced comedy with a cast of twenty-two. This was akin to running an ICU alone on the night shift. I knew I no longer wanted to be on the sidelines—I was ready to try center stage. I auditioned and was cast in a Christopher Durang play about a dysfuntional family, my introduction to the concept of co-dependency. Over the next few years I was cast in other plays. Some comedies and some poignant dramas, they all provided insight into human behavior and the power of live theater. At the urging of fellow actors who enjoyed my funny nursing stories, I started doing stand-up comedy. I dealt with the hecklers by first thinking of them as a few surgeons I knew, then let my responses fly. Each stage entrance was scary. But with each risk taken, I found I had survived relatively intact. Reinforced by dozens of self-help books, I embarked on more risk taking and slowly discovered a newfound sense of confidence and self-esteem.

Then an attorney hired me as an expert witness on a case—I made $450 for one day in court. Another attorney asked me to review and summarize some medical records. I was to be paid directly for my work; I no longer had to depend on a physician to be paid! My new company, MedicoLegal Research Services, was born. I developed a computerized format for organizing records and creating chronologies for complex personal injury and malpractice cases. Although occasionally providing medical management consultation, the bulk of my business centered on the review of medical records and the preparation of summaries and settlement demand reports.

I rapidly became a businesswoman. I had stationery, business cards, and a sample format printed; then I wrote a plan, set up books, purchased insurance plans, and hit the streets to promote my company. I soon had more business than I could handle, so I hired subcontractors to help with the typing and overload. I missed direct patient contact, yet I was making good money, and the best part—I could schedule my own hours! Within two years I had a steady clientele, was still acting in theater, and was enjoying the benefits of being my own boss. I bought a new car, new computer equipment, and eventually my dream purchase of a new ocean kayak.

Then one day my kayak, a six-foot wave and I had an argument. The wave won. I injured my back and was unable to work. Grateful that I had purchased an expensive self-employed disability insurance plan, I filed a claim. Flat on my back with sciatica, I thought I heard that wave crashing through my living room when a sheriff arrived at my front door with a subpoena. I was being sued by the insurance company to rescind my policy. They said that they would not have insured me if they had known my health history, which I had revealed completely on my application. Standard practice for many insurers is "post-claim investigation," permitted in the fine print on any claims filed within two years of purchase of the plan. I had to countersue and stepped into the dark abyss of the legal twilight zone. I wondered if it was a sort of karmic comeback *gotcha*!

The next two years were a nightmare of legal procedures and high personal costs. I returned to work full-time within eight weeks of my injury, but focused most of my consulting with a small number of attorneys who could guarantee me consistent work. In retrospect, this desire for simplification was a mistake—as an entrepreneur it is important to diversify to avoid dependence.

I became enmeshed in my own legal probelms, doing the paralegal work on my own case and allowing my business to just "survive." Other nurses were starting up their own business, and the competition was gaining on me. I had strayed from my business plan. I had become too dependent on too few attorneys, working home alone everyday—just my computer and piles of records. I was having trouble making financial ends meet and was an emotional wreck. I settled my own case in 1990 for a small amount so I could get it over with and go on with my life.

I continued taking cases at the local rate of $40 per hour, working at home. The attorneys rejected a price hike, threatening to go to my competition. Then I discovered that one of the attorneys was quadruple-billing the clients —in my name. He had been making a fortune off of me. Suddenly that old burnout prescription was refilled, and the feelings were all too familiar. I was angry, but this time unwilling to fight back. This time, the clown felt like a fool and no longer thought it could.

I was tired of working in isolation. I had become too immersed in it all; I could not maintain detachment in my legal work. I had no purpose. Deja-vu was pushing me, and I was pushing forty. I was overweight, smoking again, out of shape, and dating a jerk. Exhausting. But all that seemed relatively minor when I discovered a breast lump. Biopsy revealed it was only an abcess. I was ecstatic. Spared. My doctor prescribed antibiotics and a rest.

Instead of Tahiti, this time I went to Kauai for brief vacation and to think things out. I developed a short-term plan to help me find new long-term goals. I would spend my last few months of thirty-something in a strict training program. My short-term goal; to kayak and camp along Kauai's Na Pali coast on my fortieth birthday.

In training for forty, I followed a rigid exercise regimen of jogging and kayaking, worked to overcome my co-dependent ways and nicotine addiction, dropped my junk food habits and twenty-two pounds, got out of my dying business and my deadend relationship, painted T-shirts to sell, and wrote in my journal to rediscover my creative spirit.

I tried not to beat myself up for ignoring my business. Was I a failure as a nurse entrepreneur? I knew that the French noun *entrepreneur* was masculine and meant "contractor." That didn't sound much like nursing me. But I found both the English and French versions of the word *entrepreneur* actually came from the French verb *entreprendre*, meaning "to undertake, to take in hand, to contract for, to attempt." I found solace in realizing that being an entrepreneur is based on one's attitude and willingness to undertake a business or enterprise, not necessarily at whether one succeeds at such an attempt. Being an entrepreneur is actually a state of mind. And I was still somewhat in that altered state. But I wasn't sure any longer where I was about nursing.

I considered rebuilding my legal business, but felt that I needed more power to have control over my work. I had the Alexander Gudonov complex—feeling that I wasn't good enough. Like a nurse who constantly toys with becoming a doctor even though she dislikes medicine, I investigated law schools. I even went so far as to sit for the law school admissions test. I knew being a lawyer wasn't for me halfway through the exam when the proctor told me that if I laughed out loud one more time, I would be asked to leave. I didn't want to learn how to think like a lawyer. I had found that the legal business had nothing to do with what was right or wrong—only with what was the written law. My experiences in legal work for the past five years had been exciting only when I was dealing specifically with medical issues, not the law. I let it go.My road-to-forty regimen was paying off. I was healthy and strong. I continued to take in a few medical-legal cases to pay my bills. I still wasn't sure what I wanted to do, yet felt encouraged by having started to figure out what I didn't want. To prepare for my birthday trip, I made a trial run paddling down the Na Pali coast in June of 1990. That trip was flawless—a wonderful adventure.

I felt empowered and expected an even better time for my birthday trip. I thought I was well prepared. What I didn't account for was a scorpion in my scivvies...

It was August of 1990 with record-breaking heat in Kauai. I invited four friends to join me. We paddled with frigate birds into open sea caves and past sea turtles on our way down the coast. Our Kalalau campsite was next to a waterfall and overlooked the beach. For four days, we lazed on hammocks under trees full of singing birds. Paradise. We had my afternoon birthday party on the beach and then relaxed in the warm sunset. That evening we packed our belongings. We planned to leave early the next morning and paddle further down the coast.

Everyone else was sleeping on the beach. I was feeling fine with forty as I finished packing my gear and searched through my bags for a change of clothes. Under the shooting stars, I put on a clean T-shirt and panties. The pain was so sudden and so severe, I thought I had been shot. Twice. I ripped off my underware, but it was too dark to see what had bitten me—once in the abdomen, once in the groin. I broke out in a sweat, had diarrhea, and started vomiting. Trying not to panic, I ran to the waterfall to soak in the icy water. Within an hour I felt better. I returned to my gear, examined the two large red lumps, and then felt enormous fatigue. I lay on the ground and went to sleep.

Early the next morning, my friends woke me and asked why I hadn't come down to the beach. I didn't know. As we loaded our gear into the kayaks, I casually mentioned to one friend that something had bitten me and that it itched.

It was "kona" weather—very hot, no waves, and no wind. The ocean looked like glass, reflecting the cloudless sky. We paddled together for about two hours, then my friends went into a cove to check out a beach. I was enjoying watching the dozens of sea turtles that were swimming around them and told them I'd keep paddling towards our destination of Miloli'i, a remote camping beach accessible only by boat.

I paddled further down the coast, enjoying the tropic birds. I was watching schools of fish in the clear water around me. I remember starting to feel confused about what direction to paddle. Eskimos call it *kayak angst*, when the still waters can confuse your orientation. I stopped paddling and heard some noise. Suddenly I was surrounded by hundreds of dolphins. As I paddled, they swam along side. Every so often, one porpoise would nudge my kayak, pushing me towards the direction of shore. Mesmerized by the sounds of their breaths, I did not know how long I was with them. I remember thinking that I was in such good shape that I wasn't even sweating despite how hard I was paddling. I went to take a drink and found that my water bottle was empty. I didn't remember drinking it. That one porpoise kept rubbing against my kayak, repeatedly pushing my bow towards the shore. The dolphins swam away as I neared the channel where one of my friends was paddling in. That is the last clear memory I have of the next three days.

I don't remember landing. My friends later said that on shore, I was acting angry and told them I wanted to be alone. I vaguely recall thinking that I was telling them that I needed water and couldn't understand why they didn't help me. I remember thinking that I had to go find some water, so I walked to the other side of the mile-long beach. I don't know how long I was there, or what I was doing. I do remember falling, landing face first on the sand and being unable to move. I felt disconnected from my body. I was unable to talk. My eyes were open, but everything went from color to black and white. Funny, I did not panic. I just prayed. Then I must have lost consciousness.

A tourist found me passed out under a tree. She got my friends, who threw me in the shower and gave me water. Over the next three days, I drifted in and out of rational behavior, my friends urging me repeatedly to drink water. I remember spending a lot of time in the outhouse suffering from repeated bouts of diarrhea. They said that at times I was quite lucid, other times irritable and depressed. I thought I was asking for help. They said I never did. My friends, none of them of a medical background, later explained that they thought that it was just recurrent dehydration. My perceptions were distorted, but I could not explain it.

Once back to civilization, I could not remember landmarks or street names. Medical tests revealed an electrolyte imbalance and an allergic response, along with severe bradycardia and hypotension. It took several more weeks for doctors to put it all together. There had been a cumulative effect: allergic reaction to a scorpion sting, dehydration, heat injury, and mild encephalitis. I was frequently told how lucky I was to be alive. And I knew it. I still have a slight problem with short-term memory, but otherwise the brain is intact.

One other thing occurred during my recuperation. About two weeks after this whole experience, I saved the life of a two-year-old drowning victim. That event made me want to return to nursing.

Needless to say, I learned a lot from the entire experience. The first was gratitude. The second was grace. Third, although I wanted to exercise like I was eighteen, I had to remember that I was doing it in a forty-year-old body! From now on, I view getting old as a privilege. Fourth, all my whining and complaining and anger over the years for all the things that had gone wrong were getting me nowhere. If I needed help, I had to ask for it directly and clearly. I had to find out what I wanted and be clear on getting it. And I could no longer expect anyone else to know what I needed. My life depended on it.

Fifth, having my own business in the medical-legal field may have been economically rewarding as a nurse entrepreneur, but I wasn't happy doing it anymore. Quitting was akin to failure, and I didn't need any excuses, physical or otherwise, to change my mind. Although re-opening my business might have been the right thing to do, it was not right for me. Sixth, I wanted to work as a nurse again, get my skills back, and enjoy the positive aspects that come from helping others.

Seventh, a good sense of humor once again had pulled me through. I wanted to learn more about the healing aspects of humor and utilize that in self-care education. Eighth, I enjoyed working as a consultant, yet I wanted more power and authority to be autonomous. Ninth, I had a wealth of knowledge to be shared. Not only my professional expertise, but my experiences with insurance companies, drug companies, doctors, and lawyers as well. And tenth, I wanted to continue in my creative pursuits, including the performing arts.

So, now I'm full-time in a doctoral program in Public Health, researching everything about humor and health. I'm working part-time as a nurse practitioner and loving it. I'm clear on my boundaries now, knowing when to say no and when to ask for help. I don't give till I'm empty. I don't judge my value as a nurse on whether my patients change or what others think. I'm much more in the moment, and find I am a better nurse for it. Without the extraneous mind-babble ("good enough," anger, etc.), I'm more focused and the job is easier.

Funny, my entrepreneurial skills came into play when I took the job. I'm working at a hospital that has never used nurse practitioners or clinical nurse specialists, only physician assistants. I was able to use my business skills and sense of self-value to negotiate a new job category, a higher pay scale, flexible hours, my own perks and benefits, and have opened the door for other advanced practice nurses.

I still take a few small medical-legal cases to supplement my income. I'm doing stand-up comedy routines for business conferences and company meetings, sort of tailor-made "roasts." I'm running and paddling again and feel a strong sense of "porpoise." I'm still painting T-shirts to sell. I'm still the clown, but not the fool—reminding me that I know I can

So, I am still a nurse entrepreneur, as I'll never stop trying. I'll keep attempting new enterprises. And I'm very proud to be a nurse. At the hospital, a lot of nurses talk with me about their ideas; I'm becoming a role model and sounding board for risk takers. I encourage all nurses to expand their horizons. Nurses are unique in their capabilities. But, nurses are the only ones that don't know how talented they are. Our training and work experience has prepared us for just about anything. We're educators, advocates, professionals, technicians, counselors, administrators, healers, artists, scientists, etc.,etc. Only our frustrations, anger, tendency for co-dependency, and fears stand in our way.

I've heard the complaints of, "I don't have the expertise," or "I need the job structure," or "I don't really want my own business, I just want to do something else." No one ever readily admits how damn scared they are. They want to pass the buck, fearful that the buck would stop with them. They are afraid to take responsibility for their own lives, probably attributable to a low self-esteem. Perfectionists feel their value is based on what they do, rather than who they are. Nurses, the ultimate perfectionists, are often afraid to risk starting their own businesses for fear of failure. They think that making any mistake is a reflection of their self-worth, that they would be bad. The true joy in entrepreneurship is in the trying, in making and learning from the mistakes, and in the journey. The real payoff is self-love.

I've had enough crazy things occur in my life to know there is no such thing as security. A close friend was a nurse in San Francisco who had a medical-legal consulting business. Quite successful, he continued running it even after he discovered he had AIDS. He had the ultimate "yes, but" when he took the risk of leaving his secure staff nursing job to get his business going well. He never looked back, the business was successful, and he died knowing that he had nothing to regret.

I certainly don't recommend getting caught in legal tangles to finance a business. You can start slow, just a few hours a week while still working on your job. There will always be reasons not to do it. Don't focus on the obstacles; focus on the goals. Keep the goals clear, yet flexible. As business picks up—and it will, because nurses that can handle a floor of patients will be successful in whatever they try if they believe in themselves—start taking more risks. Feel your fears, and then risk it anyway. Consider half-time. Seek resources in the community like the SBA, the NNBA, and the library to help you along the way.

Keep a journal on your journey. Get to know and love yourself.

External work, such as business plans, are necessary. But internal changes are required, too. A paradigm shift must occur. Gather infomation to help you discard old values while embracing new ones. Keep track of what your new values and goals are. Don't stand in your own way about what should be. Remember: *you can be right, or you can be happy.*

One more point. Nurses are traditionally "rescuers." They are highly skilled at helping everyone but themselves, then wonder why they burn out and feel so angry. I think many nurses come from dysfunctional families. Rescuing is a learned behavior that helps the child survive in a stressful setting. One learns not to ask for help if one is never going to get it. One responds by giving what one needs most. But those childhood behaviors don't work in the adult world. To be successful as a nurse entrepreneur, those co-dependency ways have to be overcome. Waiting for others to change, or help you, or support you, or believe in you before you help yourself isn't the answer. You have to be your own cheerleader up those hills, chanting that you *think you can.* The answers to what you really want and how to get it are all in you. If you can dream it, you can do it. After discovering what you want, start gathering infomation to find out what you need so that you can get what you want. Extra guidance and self-trust can be gained from a few self-help books and/or supportive counseling. Learn to ask directly for what you need. Be realistic in your expectations, especially with whom you ask. Don't wait for certain people to change. Don't wait for the system to change. And don't wait for the stresses to change. I repeatedly hear, "Well, when such and such happens, then I'll be able to do it." You cannot change the stress—but you have the power to change your response to it.

Empowerment is the key to nurse entrepreneurship. Your *porpoise,* nudging you in the right direction, is within. Become quiet and listen. Don't let the calmness cause angst. Become centered, empowered, and make the mind-shift to be ready to risk.

Don't wait for a scorpion to change your mind.

UPDATE 1997

It has been a long journey with a few unexpected detours over the past six years, but I just graduated and am now a Doctor of Public Health. As planned, I spent the first few years of doctoral study learning everything I could about humor and health. My background in the performing arts was helpful in the development of my new business as a humor consultant. Now, I frequently give humor presentations, including one called "Lighten Up, Seriously!" to nurses and other health professionals, teachers, emergency workers, patients, businesses, and at large conferences. New opportunities to incorporate humor in my work arise each day. For example, I will soon teach a graduate level course in Health Promotion and Education and look forward to exploring humor strategies with the students.

Fortunately, there have been no more scorpions. However, I did experience another surprise of nature—a natural disaster—that led to amazing new directions of study and creative opportunites. It started in 1992 when a research opportunity literally blew into town. Hurricane Iniki, with winds over 145 mph, completely devastated the island of Kauai and I became intensely involved in disaster relief work.Humor was pervasive among the Iniki survivors on Kauai, which I recorded in cartoon format over a one year period of disaster recovery. These disaster -related cartoons were the catalyst for my dissertation research on "Survivor Humor in Disasters." My exploratory investigation looked at the phenomenon of Survivor Humor as a coping mechanism and positive adaptive response to disasters and crisis.

I have attended conferences and taken training courses in disaster relief work and disaster mental health services. I have also developed as a cartoonist, and have had over 50 of my editorial cartoons published in newspapers and journals in the past four years.

My company, MedicoLegal Research Services, has remained a primary source of financial support while in school. As the legal climate has changed, I have recently expanded into new directions, ie., working with physicians on research, manuscript preparation, and editing for publication. Training in computer technologies has improved my research capabilities and value as a consultant.

For right now, I'll continue with my research business, teaching, and humor consultant work. I am taking some time after graduation to relax a bit, recover financially, and explore new options. The intensive dissertation work, especially in the past year, was primarily a left-brained pursuit. Now, it's time for a little right brain action, ie., theater, kayaking, drawing, reading books I don't have to remember, travel, etc. I will eventually publish more about my research, but I have also started attending some writers' conferences. I want to learn more about writing—not just for academia, but also for fun and profit.

I have been so inspired working with disaster survivors. Despite overwhelming adversity, they sought not to endure just to survive, but to thrive. An attitude of gratitude and an ability to see the absurdity in the adversity has kept me faithful to my porpoise. I maintain a willingness to change, risk, and keep learning—which provides the impetus to seek new directions, entrepreneurial opportunities, and creative pursuits.

MedicoLegal Research Services
1532-A Anuhea Place
Honolulu, HI 96816
(808) 737-4929

Chapter 41

From Dream to Reality Through Caring

by Kate Walters, RN

Cruising at 30,000 feet somewhere over the midwestern region of the United States, the idea that I could start my own private duty home care business evolved into the beginning of a plan.

My friend and I had just quit our jobs at a home care agency that fell far short of its ideals and left us searching for a better way to live *our* ideals in home care administration. We were on our way to visit another friend who had left the same organization a few months earlier.

While in flight, I began reading the book *Starting and Operating a Business in Michigan*. The first section dealt with preliminary considerations and included a self-evaluation checklist for going into business. After completing the checklist, I was encouraged by the fact that my responses indicated that I probably had what it takes to run a business. The major factors were a willingness to forego compensation for up to five years and to plan on working sixty to eighty hours a week! My friend and I discussed the possibilities off and on while we enjoyed one anothers' company along with the sunshine of Southern California. The trip served to refresh me and to free me from the shackles of my previous jobs. I returned home determined to investigate the procedures for getting started.

In the months that followed, I sent for federal and state information on the steps to take to start a business, using Jenkins' and Lang's book as a guide. I also continued to reflect on the problems I had encountered in the organizations that I had worked for previously. Having the time to think and read was a gift, granted to me by my family who could manage without my income for awhile.

In analyzing my past experiences, the things that bothered me the most were the lack of responsiveness and commitment to both clients and field staff in private duty home care. Power struggles and profits, rather than the provision of quality services, seemed to be the primary forces for action. Field staff were underpaid, undertrained, and usually underappreciated. This was not a problem unique to my experiences. A demonstration project funded by the Ford Foundation highlighted some of the work-life issues of the homemaker/home health aide.

In this study, wage levels, benefits, and opportunities for advancement were identified as major issues—with part-time, episodic work, training and support emerging as minor issues impacting on the recruitment and retention of homemaker/home health aides. Work-life improvement projects were then undertaken, and those projects did show improvement in retention and satisfaction among workers. Unfortunately, when the funding for the projects were withdrawn, most of the work-life improvements were not continued by the agencies involved in the study. Belief in the value of the work-life improvements, both for the worker and the clients served, was not powerful enough in itself to motivate these organizations to initiate change.

It is my belief that having satisfied workers with decreased turnover will also result in satisfied clients—and increased profits in the long run. The challenge for the industry and for me was to place quality of work-life and quality care at the forefront, and to overcome the political and financial barriers to change. I was sure that there could be a better way to do this business that would focus on *care* of clients and stafff and also maintain profitability. But first, let me explain what this service is all about.

Private duty home care is long-term care service, usually paid for out-of- pocket, by which individuals receive assistance with self-care needs that enables them to maintain their independence and stay at home. Although family members continue to provide for many of these needs, outside services are increasingly needed since our older population is growing, and many adult children of the elderly are working themselves.

What these individuals and families need is someone they can turn to who understands the problems they are facing, and who will be able to provide the expertise and the people to resolve those problems. Responsiveness to this need requires training, commitment, and certainly caring. I firmly believe that nurses have the most appropriate training for evaluating and planning the long-term care of our aging and chronically-ill population. But nurses can't do it alone!

Clients don't usually need the level of care that nurses are trained for—except for the evaluation, planning, and supervision of that care. Often neglected but very important people in this scenario are the homemaker/home health aides, or as we call them, the Home Support Assistants. A successful private duty home care agency therefore must be concerned about care for the clients, while caring for the individuals who provide services for those clients. Care must become the central focus of both client services and staff relations.

The words *care* and *caring* have been a part of nursing from the beginning, but the terms have been used without real inquiry into their meaning until recently. Caring is seen as an essential component of human survival in this world—and nursing, by focusing on this concept and developing its meaning, has great potential power for change in healthcare and in society.

Caring is defined by Mayeroff as "helping another to grow and to actualize oneself." Caring assumes continuity, for caring is a developmental process. Nursing administrators are in a pivotal position to either promote caring, or to lose it within the present confusion about power and politics in the highly structured environment of the healthcare system. Within the private duty sector of home care, a greater potential exists for developing a home care service that is responsive to the needs of each client and each caregiver, if only we would dare to try. Convinced that it could and should be done, the next step involved was finding out just how to accomplish it.

With the help of a lawyer friend, I found out what legal procedures needed to be followed to open a business. In Michigan, to open this type of business as a sole proprietorship, all that was needed was to register in the county as a DBA (doing business as) and pay a fee (of course). That part was easy! Next came the big questions: Where would the money come from to finance the start-up? Where to locate? How long we could operate on start-up money?

The whole process gained momentum when two things happened. First, the *I* became a *we* when a friend who had worked with me at the previous agency decided to become a part of this endeavor. The second thing that pushed us forward was the approval of a home equity loan on my house for start-up money for the business.

Before going any further, I had to confront my family with the risks and the real and potential financial sacrifices that this move entailed. I had to be sure that they were with me all the way, because I knew it was not going to be easy. They assured me that they thought it was great and that they could handle it.
Even though I knew there would be days when we all would long for a little hot dog stand on the corner, their support and my friend's involvement provided the impetus to take the leap.

Over the next several weeks, my partner and I met with vendors for the equipment we would need and searched for an office. We had already decided on the general location by identifying an area of the country that was not serviced adequately by existing agencies. Once we found suitable office space, the momentum picked up again.

Some of those early activities were fun and, of course, some were frustrating. Meeting with vendors and sales people was a real challenge, since we had to sound like we knew what we were doing while seeking information from them. What we found, through, was that we went into those meetings much more prepared than many of the sales people. We began to get real picky about who we would even talk to, and for the most part we were able to connect with honest people who really wanted to help us. Our meetings took place at my house until we had the office, and then we met at one table in an otherwise empty space. We have pictures of the office from those days, and the room that we met in is now the "hub" of our business with four desks, two tables, a copy machine, a fax, and walls covered with maps and message boards.

Besides meeting with sales people, we also shopped for furniture which we purchased from a membership warehouse and hauled and assembled ourselves. We were able to adequately furnish the office for around $1,200, a significant savings compared to any office supply store. Another way that we saved money was by tapping into the skills and talents of family and friends. My brother assisted me in the purchase of a computer and software for word processing and data collection, and is still working with us on computerization of our scheduling and accounting system. Without him, I would have been lost in the maze of computer technology.

My sister also helped by getting me started with payroll since I knew nothing about the FICA, FUTA, SUTA lingo of payroll. I remember calling my sister when I tried to do the first payroll and realized that I didn't have the state tax tables in the plethora of information I had received from the Michigan Ombudsman's office. She talked me through the first payroll, and now does my weekly payroll on her computer while we work on setting up our own systems on our computer.

Our first client was also a memorable experience! We had been working on the development of our documentation record systems when we received a call for assistance in caring for a terminally-ill client. I was still working part-time at a local hospital, and my partner contacted me there to tell me about the case. As I was driving up to the office, I realized that we didn't even have the paperwork ready to do the assessment! I went into a panic as we threw something together from the forms we were working on. I then tried to calm myself. I have assessed hundreds of clients before, but this was *our* first client, and I was nervous. Then the client died in just a few days, and the family came in to pay the bill before I had even set up a way to bill for services! This experience was yet another catalyst for moving forward with setting up systems for handling the work, and it brought the dream into clearer focus.

Work continued to come in slowly in response to several methods we used to advertise. We notified friends and associates through printed announcements and phone calls; we sent out coupons for introductory discounts through a blanket mailing to selected zip codes, and we did some spot ads on a local radio station. Many days were spent waiting for the phone to ring, and when it did, my partner would say "business!" in the hopes that it would be a new client. I told him that there would come a time when we would relish those quiet days when we could work on forms and spend extra time with the staff and clients. That day has arrived!

In our second year we incorporated—and significantly increased revenues to the point where we could even see the possibility of *paying* our administrator. We have had days when a hot dog stand seemed like a better idea, but overall we are proud of our accomplishments, and we look forward to expanding by opening satellite offices in nearby communitites where we have identified the same lack of available services that brought us to this community.

We believe that caring is the most important element in our relationship with our staff and in their work with the clients. We can teach people how to perform tasks; we can't teach them how to care. We can only foster that caring by taking care of *one another* while we provide care for our clients. I know we have failed sometimes in living this ideal, and we will sometimes fail again because we are all human, and we make mistakes. If our belief in caring as the central focus of our organization continues to guide our actions, we will succeed in fulfilling our dream. I also believe that we all will make a fair living doing it.

Looking back over the first two years, I believe that our rapid growth was due largely to the trust that other people in the community already had in us—and that we did not disappoint them when they referred cases to us. The timing was right for us to start this agency when we did, but it left me with some unfinished business (such as my thesis!) that was very difficult to find time for when the work load became heavy.

At each phase of the business development there were steps that were unfamiliar to us, and we had to turn to other people or to the library for help. This kind of learning-as-you-go can be slow and painful, so it is a good thing that we understood the day-to-day basics of this business before we started. In fact, I think that the most important first step in starting a nursing business is to really *know* the business you are going to start. Not only should you know that business, you need to like it! For some people this knowing and liking may develop over a period of time, and new ideas will develop from patience in the learning.

We believe our future is strong, and we are looking forward to new ventures anc activities that we haven't begun to dream of yet. We care for the very *human* people who make up our organization, which in turn promotes caring service to our clients. This is our greatest strength that will carry us through to the future!

References

1Jenkins, M.D. & Lang, T.O. (1986). *Starting and Operating a Business in Michigan.* Milipitas, CA: Oasis Press.
2 Feldman, P.H. with Sapienca, A.M. & Kane, N.M. (1988) *Who Cares for Them? Workers, Work Life Problems and Reforms in the Home Care Industry.* Cambridge, MA: Dept. of Health & Policy Management, Harvard School of Public Health.
3 Mayeroff, M. (1971). *On Caring.* NY: Harper & Row.

UPDATE 1997

Caring Home Support Services, Inc. is alive and well but much has changed since we last talked. Yes, it's true that partnerships are...well, *a pain* and the person that started out with me has been gone for over five years. The leaving was not easy and much was learned in the process. Yes, it is also true that having employees is...well, *a pain*, but again we have learned much and now we have a smaller staff than a couple of years ago but we are mightier than ever!!

We have grown as a community of people who *really care* about one another and who really care about the work that we do. Our financial growth has been flat over the past couple of years, and you know what? That is *just fine* with me. Growth is not worth it if it means hiring too fast to keep up with the work and then having to fire just as fast when the people hired in haste don't work out. I am much happier with no or slow growth and doing our absolute best while nurturing and, yes, loving one another. We have the *best* Home Care Aides supported in their good work by the kindest, most caring office staff I have ever had the pleasure to work with.

Recently I received an award as one of Michigan's Top Nurses of

1996. The focus of this award was my work as a servant leader. The true test of servant leadership is whether or not those led grow as persons, become healthier and freer, and become more likely themselves to serve. It is most important to me how well I have done on this test. I am thrilled that this award indicates that, perhaps, I *am* making significant progress.

So, where are we now? What have we learned? Where are we going?

With the dramatic changes in the homecare marketplace, I know that to survive and continue to do good work, we need to affiliate with another organization that offers the other home care services. My soul-work belongs with supporting and nurturing Home Care Aides, but stand-alone private duty companies are perhaps a thing of the past. I don't believe that it is for the better but I do believe it is what is happening.

We have learned that working with people is challenging, frustrating, and extremely rewarding. I believe that we have achieved our goal of having a core, a dedicated team of Home Care Aides who stick with us through the good and bad times. Our average length of employment of our current staff is 4 years. This is NOT a common occurrence in this type of business.

I have learned that I love being a business owner, so, of course, I am starting another business called Care Works, Inc. The focus of this business is finding businesses that truly care in all aspects of business life and then helping busy people connect with these great, caring companies. Are there enough of them out there? I certainly hope so. There are other aspects of Care Works but we are still in the early development stages of that company.

Our goals remain the same, to provide a great work environment that truly and wholly supports the good work of Home Care Aides. Now we have to find a way to do that as part of a larger organization. Through Care Works, we are also refining our education programs for Home Care Aides and plan to market our works to other great organizations. We are also looking at ways to continue our efforts to support workers and improve workers' health, sometimes in spite of the workplace, since I am very concerned about the effect of work on our health and our spirits.

Do I regret what I did? Heck no! Do I think more nurses should start their own businesses? You bet!! Through the Michigan Nurses in Business, I and my fellow nurse entrepreneurs endeavor to empower Michigan nurses to be entrepreneurial in their work and to create wholeness in their lives through:

* Skill building
* Mentoring
* Networking
* Providing a link with other resources
* Identifying business opportunities
* Promoting self-care
* Nurturing self confidence and self esteem
    (*Mission statement of the Michigan Nurses in Business*)

I am also developing a Certificate program in Nurse Entrepreneurship for Madonna University. I truly believe that starting businesses is a vital pathway for promoting the profession of nursing and for promoting the economic and professional growth of nurses. But, nurses need more business savvy. NNBA, MNBA and soon, the Certificate program are significant parts of this process.

Caring Home Support Services, Inc.
3093 Sashabaw
Waterford, MI 48329
(810) 673-9820
Fax: (810) 673-9828

Chapter 42

It is Not the Critic
Who Counts

by Janice M. Stanfield, RN, CETN

Becoming a nurse had always been a dream for me. I was excited at the prospect of making a *real* contribution to society.

I spent the first six years of my career in critical care, working day after day in life and death situations. It was very exciting, and I felt I was contributing so much. But soon, I became the expert at "how to"...how to calibrate a Swan Ganz, how to assist with a pacemaker insertion, how to fix just about any piece of machinery that was broken. I found myself working odd hours, all days of the week. I no longer felt fulfilled. I had become a technician. I was no longer working with conscious patients; personal interactions were a thing of the past.

Family life, what was that? When I wasn't sleeping or working, my son was asleep and my husband at work. My dream had become a nightmare. In 1978, after fighting ulcerative colitis throughout my second pregnancy, I was readmitted with the disease completely out of control. They wanted to do a permanent ileostomy. Stool, uncontrollably seeping through a hole in the abdomen... how appalling! As a nurse, I didn't seem to warrant the same explanations given a lay person. My brother died of complications acquired during the same surgery for the same disease. As a critical care nurse, all I ever saw was suffering, discomfort, and sometimes death—certainly without dignity—when it came to patients with the same diagnosis. Quality of life had to mean something, so I refused the operation.

Harrassed night and day by surgeons and my own husband, who threw his wedding ring at me in anger, threatening to divorce me if I didn't consent to the surgery, the struggle against pain and fear lost out. In August of 1978, I awakened in intensive care with an ileostomy. I felt beaten. I had lost.

One day, shortly before my discharge from the hospital, a woman came in. She identified herself as an enterostomal therapy nurse. I was a nurse, yet I had never heard of that specialty. She briefly showed me how to put onto my abdomen a long, clear bag to catch the stool. It looked terrible. I was uncomfortable, and I thought I carried an odor everyplace I went. Why didn't they let me die? Who wants to live like this? But the disease was gone; I was going to live. It seemed I had no more choices. I was going to live whether I liked it or not, so I had better get my life back together again. In October of 1978, I was discharged home to a family I no longer knew—a child of four that I had not seen in months and a baby I had not had the chance to get to know.

I had been unemployed for months. I was trying to recover from a serious illness, trying to recapture some personal worth and improve my body image. Shortly after I arrived home my husband walked out. He couldn't handle the stress. He said I had failed him. Left with thousands of dollars in debt, in grief over loss of identity, my role as a wife, employment as a nurse, and my body image, I wallowed in self-pity. No one understood my cry for help. I alienated every friend I ever had. It seemed I had failed at everything I tried to do.

Then, in April of 1980, a truly wonderful friend came into my life. He had faith in me. He helped me to realize that I could turn all my adversity into triumph if I would just alter my goals. Why not become an enterostomal therapy nurse? After all, there is nothing like first-hand experience. So, my new goal? Make a substantial contribution...become the best that I could be, make a diffrnece in someone's life. My friend became my husband; he supported my return to school by assisting with the care of my children and assisting financially and emotionally. In December, I graduated from the Cosler School of Enterostomal Therapy at the University of Southern California.

Enterostomal therapy, being a fairly new field of nursing at that time, had not yet earned its place among budgeted staff in the hospital setting. It rapidly became clear to me that if I wanted to pursue this line of nursing, my only choice was independent practice.

I contacted numerous insurance companies, posing as a potential subscriber, to determine how the service was reimbursed, and at what rate. I learned that in order to provide the service, my patient had to be referred by a physician, and either seen in a hospital, at home or in a physician's office. General health visits were not covered. Therefore, there was no need for me to obtain office space; I could set up an office in my home.

I purchased business cards, Roladex cards, and obtained a digital pager, a business phone line and a 24-hour answering service. Over the next ten months, my husband set up a computer system and customized a patient management system which allowed me to document according to Medicare guidelines in record time. He set up an automated billing system, eliminating the need for outside secretarial and billing services, and cut my overhead by 75 percent.

I marketed to physicans, hospitals and home health agencies, and set up numerous contracts to provide my services as needed. This proved to be most cost-effective for the client, eliminating the need to hire a full-time, or even a part-time employee for services needed only occasionally. I obtained my BRN Provider number and offered one free hour of continuing education to the agencies and hosptials for each twenty new patient referrals. Not only did this thrill the client, but always following my inservices, I had an increase in patient referrals. It kept me busy full-time doing what I loved most, helping ostomates to understand that they are not alone, that there are many resources for them, and helping them regain their full potential, and get on with a quality life. I was truly fulfilled.

As the ET nurse role expanded to include wound and dermal ulcer care, so did my practice. Patient load increased, and I found the need to subcontract visits to other ET nurses. Now service areas are well defined, which decreases time on the road and increases profit margins.

Three years into the business, when my gross reached six figures, we moved to a larger home ten miles closer to my service area. Reimbursement policies were still unchanged, so I found the expense of an outside office remained unnecessary. I purchased a car for the company, added a cellular phone, copy machine, modem line, and updated my computer system. My patient files were transferred to floppy disks and stored in a 12" x 15" fireproof safe, thereby eliminating the need for excessive storage space.

Today my company, Stanfield Associates, Enterostomal Therapy Nurse Consultants, is thriving. We see ostomy patients in hospitals, set them up with suppliers, and arrange dressing and ostomy equipment deliveries for home care follow-up. We manage their care to optimal functrioning, and after discharge we are always available to them for questions or recurring problems.

We work as consultants in wound management, evaluating pressure relief devices and suggesting updated management methods, thereby decreasing costs both in product and nursing visits needed. We "revamp" central supply departments, eliminating outdated equipment and assisting in cost savings for hospitals. Policy and procedure manual review, in relation to our field of expertise, is also a service we offer. Clinical research and participation in studies relating to potential products have proven to be a good source of income, and it is just plain fun, with frequent opportunities to travel.

I contract with insurance companies, who have come to realize our cost-saving systems provide the *best* quality care at the lowest possible cost, cutting the length a patient is on service by updating management methods and decreasing healing time. We have spoken to several community organizations, including the Ostomy Association, and give professional inservices at least monthly. We have served as expert witnesses and done a fair amount of chart review for medical malpractice attorneys.

I work the hours I choose, leaving home when my children leave for school and arriving home before their buses. I spend the afternoons doing paper work, special projects, making phone calls and setting up appointments for my next working day. I prepare my patients at the onset of service to handle any urgent problems independently, thereby decreasing all emergency visits to about a dozen a year.

As far as tips go, I think being organized is the most important factor in independent practice. It is a big timesaver. Also, keep in mind that you can't be afraid to make an investment in equipment which will save you time, keep you sane, and present a professional image. My initial financial investment was less than $1,800.

Lessons learned? The first thing I learned is that it is okay to ask for a fair reimbursement for my services. I think nurses often feel guilty when asking for money because it isn't the Florence Nightingale thing to do. However, employees are paid for their hours and get benefits to boot. Your rates must include your overhead—that includes life, health and disability insurance, and days off for illness or vacation. DON'T underestimate your value.

Probably the most important thing I've learned is that you have to be a self-starter. You don't make a penny or contribute anything to society by watching the morning soaps. You have to be a risk taker. You have to get out there, believe in yourself and your service, and make it happen.

Today, I couldn't be happier. Honored this year by my peers, who voted me the "Pacific Coast ET Nurse of the Year,"and by a state consumer group who recognized me as "Health Care Professional of the Decade," my goals were fulfilled. I guess it's time for some new ones—possibly a low-cost supply depot, an incontinence clinic, or getting that nursing reimbursement bill through Congress. As Registered Nurses, our opportunitites are truly endless.

I recently was visiting the office of a very dear friend, another nurse entrepreneur practicing in Northern California. I saw on her wall a quote from Theodore Roosevelt that says it all:

> It is not the critic who counts, not the one who points out how the strong man stumbled or how the doer of deeds might have done them better. The credit belongs to the one who is actually in the arean, whose face is marred with sweat and dust and blood; who strives valiantly; who errs and comes up short again; who knows the great enthusiams, the great devotions and spends himself in a worthy cause; who, if he wins, knows the triumps of high achievement; and who if he fails, at least while daring greatly, so that his place shall never be with those cold and timid souls who know neither victory no defeat.

UPDATE 1997

Five years have passed since I wrote the preceding story. The business has really flourished. I now sub-contract with three certified ET nurses, two full-time and one part-time. My husband has become my only employee. He works part-time for me, in addition to his primary job. He serves as a technical expert to assist with software development and computer management services. Since he has long contributed to the development of the technical aspects of my company, his employee status allows for better tax benefits (under the BIZ PLAN), and I put funds away at the end of each year in accounts for each of us, to prepare for retirement.

The 1994 Northridge earthquake set us back a bit, but we have since recovered. My company remains home based, however, with the huge influx of managed care here in southern California, an out patient clinic is looking more and more beneficial. I am negotiating in that arena.

We continue to be heavily involved in clinical product trials and have published several articles related to this research. The publications have assisted in generating even more business.

With two of my sons now in college in the east, my frequent travelling to lecture or participate in research meetings allows me to visit them for a nominal increase in airfares. It's wonderful having the flexibility in my schedule to make those visits.

Life is great! Busy...but great! One of my mentors once said, "You do in life what you want to do. Do it with passion, commitment and at the end of each day, look back and be proud of your day's work. If you follow your heart, career success and financial reward will just happen." She was right.

I continue to live by the meaning behind the words of President Roosevelt, which I cited in my first story. You can never be afraid to take a chance... "It's not the critic who counts..."

Stanfield & Associates
Enterostomal Therapy Consultants
23718 LaSalle Canyon Drive
Santa Clarita, CA 91321
(818) 362-6049   Fax: (818) 255-6421

Chapter 43

On My Own

by Mary Lou Catania, RN

There were many times when my husband would suggest starting a business. We had owned a motel and had other business ventures that we were involved in at various times, but I had no desire to go into business as a nurse.

I am basically a selfish person. I liked to work my stated number of hours and go home to my family. I avoided positions that demanded a lot of overtime.

In 1982, I was in an unfortunate work-related accident. A nursing career that I enjoyed was seemingly taken from me. It wasn't until 1986, when my husband died, that I seriously started thinking about using my nursing experience as a business career. The day Sam died our major source of income was gone. As a widow with three boys in school, I needed a paycheck.

It was in my own need for a mammogram that I began to research mammography. I came to believe that my community needed a mammography center that was accessible and affordable using state-of-the-art equipment. Our local hospital was using equipment that it had been using for fifteen years and was comfortable with that type of equipment.

My husband had always enjoyed the stock market and had done fairly well with the little money we had. Initially, I was going to sell only a part of the stock to start my business. In the ensuing months, I sold all of the stock to keep the business going.

.The Mammography Center opened, participating in the American Cancer Society project for mammography. We were extremely busy, and the physicians willingly referred patients. After several weeks there was a dramatic decrease in patient load. This was due to the pressure on physicians by the hospital not to refer to my center.

Within a few months, the Mammography Center of Monterey became the only facility in our area to be granted accreditation by the American College of Radiology. We were honored with a Small Business Award by the Chamber of Commerce, a Congressional Award, and other recognition.

The women in the community have been very supportive. Business is improving every month. It has taken a lot of hard work and many, many hours. I have had to learn that one needs to be out in the community as much as possible to be seen. I realized the importance of advertising and marketing a new business. I neglected to budget adequately for advertising. You can't open a business and hide. As a nurse educator, I give presentations to groups and offer educational programs.

It has been a difficult challenge with the hospital having done everything possible to close my doors. I have held on to the belief that if you offer a quality service, at an affordable price, you can't go wrong. Our price is considerably less than any other facility in the area for a mammogram. I accept self-referral within limitations of our clinic policies.

In my research of mammography centers, it never occurred to me that they were all physician-owned or hospital-based. No one ever suggested to me that, as a woman and a nurse, it would be difficult to start a business. I use the word "difficult," as I've learned nothing is impossible. My advice to any nurse entrepreneur would be to do your research, and if you feel strongly that there is a need, go for it!

Mammography Center of Monterey
700 Cass Street, Suite 120
Monterey, CA 03940
(408) 373-8932

Chapter 44

Openness And Flexibility:
A Nurse Entrepreneur

by Barbara Nelson Kroll, RN, BSN, MA

Successful consultants always say they can do something no matter what. Then they find someone to help them to do it right.

Because I am open and flexible to new ideas, I became a nurse entrepreneur. One summer I was working as a staff nurse in a hospital as my summer job between teaching assignments. A friend of mine telephoned: "Barb, I have this medical malpractice case that I would like you to look at." My answer: "I don't even know how to spell defendant, let alone know anything about medical malpractice." I accepted the job with assurances from my attorney friend that I would be assisted to learn what I needed to know. To gain the legal knowledge that I needed, I attended workshops, read a lot, and asked many questions.

Originally, I worked a few hours a month on the case, but eventually the trial date was approaching and I needed to spend more time in the attorney's office. To manage this, I worked less in the hospital and used school vacations from teaching to work on the claim. It wasn't long before the attorney's office was getting steady inquiries and requests to have situations evaluated for a possible claim of medical negligence against a doctor, nurse, and/or hospital.

An entrepreneur in business suggested that I become an entrepreneur and market to many attorneys. Another friend helped me create a brochure describing my business. This original list included the legal services that I could provide to attorneys:

*summaries of medical records
*interpretations of medical records
*interrogatory questions developed
*deposition questions developed
*medical research
*trial preparation assistance

Because I was an assistant professor of nursing we included:

*consulting and education on health-related issues
*design and development of educational materials

Then I developed a list of workshops that I could teach. My teenage daughters and I sat around the kitchen table to brainstorm the logo. We created a white inner line surrounding my initials—inexpensive, but attractive.

Finding a good printer who would work with me was an important first step in creating my business. Having the graphics done professionally and purchasing business cards and stationery lent credibility to my first mailings.

After sending out the brochures to my Christmas card list, my friend called with my first business. It was an omen that I didn't recognize at the time—an indictator of things to come. There would be more requests for me to speak to groups of nurses about legal problems than actual work as a medical-legal consultant.

Presenting workshops is currently the majority of my entrepreneurial business. These are delivered through community colleges and technical schools that have a commitment to providing quality continuing education to their communities. Usually the length is three to seven hours.

My experience in teaching nursing helped tremendously in putting workshops together. Another help was attending a workshop on training techniques and being a member of the local chaper of the American Society of Training and Development. All these gave me the knowledge and experience to teach to a variety of participants. Some topics that I teach are appropriate for participants other than healthcare workers. Expanding my training/teaching business to groups other than nurses is my goal. I recently had a positive experience doing customer service training to front line employees of a large service station chain.

Another facet of my business is writing. I have written twelve independent study programs, each five hours in length. This was a logical step after I had created an all-day workshop on the topic. In this way I am able to use my research in more than one way. I have also written some materials for interactive software on intravenous therapy for a software company.

After the first year, I made some money and realized that I needed an accountant. My financial papers would have been in better order if I had found one before I made any money. An accountant is a tax deductible expense who can save you money.

Currently, I balance my business with teaching at a university one semester and working part-time at a hospital. My business involves presenting up to three workshops a week, writing a lot, and occasionally consulting with attorneys. This takes enormous tolerance for multiple bits of information and continuous change.

A successful entrepreneur must practice good self-care and lead a balanced life in order to survive over the long term. Having lunch with people who are nurses, entrepreneurs, or just friends is rejuvenating and inspiring for me. Many of my best ideas have resulted from taking time to smell the flowers with my friends.

Be open to opportunity; it may appear with the next telephone call.

UPDATE 1997

Now I am an entrepreneur full time! Two years ago I quit my part-time job as a crisis intervention nurse in a busy emergency room and began working at my business full time. Flexibility continues to be the moving force necessary for success. If a potential job means that I need to learn about team building or another topic—I still say "Yes, I can do that". "Can do" is my motto. Either "I can do" or I will find someone who can help me to do it successfully. Consequently, special requests cause me to grow and learn professionally in very interesting ways.

Long ago I grew bored with being a specialist on one topic. The people who hire me like to have me come back, so I have created programs to meet their needs. Because of these requests I have developed workshops on customer service, total quality management, team building, telephone skills and infection control.

Meeting new people and exploring new issues is something that I love. Creating new workshop often interests me more than teaching the old ones. It is more time consuming, but it keeps me working for the same individuals and traveling back to the same towns over and over again. Marketing lore says it is cheaper to keep the old customers than it is to market and obtain new customers.

One topic in which I have done a lot of lecturing is documentation. After reviewing numerous medical records for attorneys, I have an idea about what is a good defensive charting. I have a message to deliver to nurses. The message broadcasts how to chart for good defense and for reimbursement purposes. Having testified in court trials I know how important the charting is to helping a nurse's memory. I vary the message by including the assessment the nurse must do before charting or talking about the telephone calls that must be documented. From this I have branched out into teaching workshops on legal and ethical issues of patient care.

This summer I traveled to San Diego, California and Norfolk, Virginia to prepare some major reports for an attorney. For fun I worked as a camp nurse at a German Language Camp. This fall I will be teaching 27 workshops, speaking at a statewide long term care conference. One hot topic is "Nursing Errors that Lead to Legal Problems." Another is on mental health issues in the elderly, or motivation, recognition and criticism of employees.

Usually I travel out of state in January and June to teach a NCLEX review course for new graduate nurses. I was stranded in Philadelphia for three days by the Blizzard of '96. I had quite an adventure waiting for the airport to open. I traveled on to Iowa arriving a day late; taught a day of class; then almost lost my composure at the airline ticket counter when they said the flight was canceled because of the weather.

Some women friends question why I like to travel. I usually tell them that it is because I get my own clicker for the television in the evening while staying at the motel. Actually it is because I enjoy meeting new people and understanding their lifestyle and their style of nursing care. But traveling means that I have to be organized with my home life so that the bills get paid, the house is cleaned and the cat is fed.

In between the traveling and speaking I am doing some writing. I write a column titled "Legal Lite" for *Nightingale News*, a mid-west publication for nurses. I have also written many independent study programs for continuing education for nurses and have created an audiotape about managing the angry customer. Much of my graduate studies involved creating educational material: paper, audiovisual and computer educational materials. Writing educational materials is enjoyable work.

Remember when you were a student? Remember how there was always one more chapter or article to read, one more list of drugs or side effects to memorize? Well, being an entrepreneur is much like that. There is always a new popular author to become familiar with, a topic to research or marketing to make. Even if all my workshops are prepared with lectures, slides and handouts in order, I can always do more marketing. So being an entrepreneur is like being a student or a teacher; you can always spend more time studying and prepping.

If I ever feel caught up on my marketing I can always spend time learning a nw program for my computer. It is nice to have computer upgrades, but why do I have to take precious time away from my business to learn it? The answer? Because I like being increasingly more productive with my time. Sometimes my time is spent deciding which machine I should purchase to improve my efficiency.

An important source of energizing for me is being active in nursing associations. It is a way to meet and network with other nurses. This allows me to bounce ideas off another professional and to learn of other interests, opinions and ideas. Some of my best material has been created over a casual lunch with a fellow nurse. It is important for the entrepreneur to stay in circulation with nurses from a variety of nursing areas.

Being a nurse entrepreneur requires infinite patience while people decide whether to hire you or not, waiting for the event you scheduled six months from now, and waiting six to eight weeks or sometimes longer for the check to actually be in the mail. It requires not being too disappointed when the event gets canceled for lack of interest or the person who hired you forgot to publicize the event. It requires that the entrepreneur satisfy many different types of customers with many different types of needs.

BNK Consultants
3045 Standridge Place
St.Paul, Minnesota 55109

Chapter 45

The Center for Nursing Excellence

(This profile appeared in the March 1990 issue of the *Nurse-Entreprenuer's Exchange*.)

Editor's Note: The Center for Nursing Excellence, founded in mid-1989, and located in Newtown, PA, offers continuing education pro grams, career counseling for nurses, and educational needs/assessment programs to health care facilities.

We interviewed Helene K. Nawrocki, RN, MSN, CNA, Center co-founder, Director of Management/Leadership Development, and Associate Marketing Director, to report on the Center's activities and rapid success—a success, in large part, due to the vision and philosophy of its five founders.

NEE: Where did the idea for the Center originate?

Helene: "In twenty years of nursing, I spent twelve to fifteen years in different management and administrative positions. In my last position I ran a nursing department, and while decentralizing and educating the staff, I realized that it was time to move out and create my own system in order for me to be as creative and productive as I could be—rather than working within the hospital system, which can be so oppressive.

So, I went out on my own in 1984, and did independent consulting working for nursing publishers doing clinical editing and writing textbooks. Other clients included community colleges and businesses, for which I provided nursing workshops and management training.

Several nurse colleagues and I began to meet last summer and started brainstorming about creating our own system, because even in working with the community colleges, we couldn't be as positive and empowering as we wished. So, by last September, the Center for Nursing Excellence was up and running; between September and the end of December we had over 700 registrants attend our programs. The Center consists of five nurse owners with varied backgrounds, so we each carry a different section of the programming that's done."

NEE: What topics are covered in your continuing education programs?

Helene: "We have everything from Empowerment, Leadership/Management, Autonomy, Assertive Communications, Networking and Mentoring, to Clowning (a humor program). We have about thirty-five nurses that also teach for us on a consulting basis. There's a group of people that do clinical programs, there is a geronotological section and an RN refresher program. We have a Bridge program that runs at several local facilities, which helps them get an eye on new employees, and helps us have a place to take people clinically.

One thing you hear is that people have less time and money, and still feel the pressure to keep up, so we are looking for some fun things; a new program I created for this spring is University on the Bus™. We'll rent a bus, and I'll present a two-hour program on Time Managment on the bus on the way to a huge shopping mall. The registrants will spend all day shopping, and then I'll do another program on the way back. They earn contact hours, network with other people, and have some fun."

NEE: How does the Center advertise its programs?

Helene: "We do direct mail brochures. Our new brochures have only been out ten days, and every two days we get a couple of new clients. We mail approximately 15,000 pieces statewide, and have plans to mail beyond the state soon."

NEE: Tell us about the Center's career counseling services.

Helene: "Nurses call in, and then meet with one of the five major players in the business on a one-to-one basis for counseling and resume preparation assistance."

NEE: What kinds of careers are nurses looking for?

Helene: "Oftentimes it starts out being more of a life-balance issue. When you get through some of the negativity and overwhelmingness that they're feeling, you get to the fact that everything's out of balance—not just the job. It becomes more a process of sorting out what they do best, what they like, and looking at how often they really get to do that in their present job. And then helping them look at perhaps other positions, or other ways to use their nursing abilities and staying in nursing, though perhaps not in acute care.

Nurses are looking for areas where they can have more autonomy and control. I think that's a retention issue that facilities are missing. They're spending lots of money on recruitment, and only the wiser ones spend money on retention. It is the decade for nursing to restructure and grab some of the power and gusto, because people don't want to leave nursing—it's the frustrations that revolve around the job, and not the job itself. I find that when you work with a disgruntled, troublesome employee, and empower them, you realize that they've got good ideas. They need someone to nurture them and facilitate their growth, instead of just putting them down all the time."

NEE: Does the Center consult with hospitals to share this philosophy with them?

Helene: "Yes. I teach management/leadership development to facilities. I typically do a twelve-to-eighteen-month contract where I do one program a month with the nurse management team. But in between that time, I'm available as a consultant for problem solving.

I also meet with the vice president and CEO every third month to let them know what I see happening, and also to run interference. Because I've found that you can get one level excited, and as soon as they spread their wings, the level above them is not comfortable with that—so they throw up walls. So, if I see the V.P. level getting uncomfortable, I work with them to get beyond that, so they're comfortable enough to let people fall and scrape their knees, if that is necessary. What happens then is that every level begins to grow. It has been very successful because it's long-term."

NEE: What's on the horizon for the Center?

Helene: "We envision a Center where nurses can come—not just for continuing education—but personal, financial, and business counseling as well. We are talking now with nurse-MBA's and psych nurses in private practice to see if they'd be willing to spend some hours at the Center providing services. Nurses that have a membership could then come and use those services.

Eventually, we'd like to franchise becasue we can't do it all, and these Centers need to be everywhere. There has to be people out there that we can connect with that have the same vision and mentality. If you trust and believe that people will become empowered and reach their potential—and give them the necessary tools—then they will. It is a great decade for nurses, and our goal is to be out there empowering as many as we can."

The Center for Nursing Excellence
Pennswood Village, Suite 6
Newtown, PA 18940
(215) 396-9110

Chapter 46

Turning Points

by Alfreda Walker, RN, MSN

The decision to enter the business world was not a difficult one for me or my partner, Joyce Weinheimer, BSN.

I was at a turning point in my career. I felt that my ability to enhance someone else's financial status was no longer my goal. Throughout my entire nursing career I had worked diligently to help achieve the goals of my employer, but I often felt that my contributions were never fully appreciated. I realized that my personal satisfaction would best be achieved by doing something for myself.

Joyce was returning from a nursing stint in Saudi Arabia in late 1985, and was also tired of the daily grind associated with managing personnel and failing to receive the recognition required for her efforts. When the idea for a service that offered centralized information to nurses was discussed, we wasted very little time in developing NurseNet.

NurseNet was officially incorporated in May of 1986 with three initial founding partners. We started the company with a total of $17,000 in personal contributions. We worked through the Small Business Development Center at Georgia State University to assist in the development of our buisness plan and hired a computer programmer to develop our database program. We started our office with the purchase of a computer, printer, basic office furnishing, and a phone with a Wats line. We sublet a small space monthly from another company.

The service initially targeted the ten southeastern states. We obtained a mailing list of 1,500 hospitals and mailed a letter to every hospital announcing the service. In addition, we selected ten hospitals in Georgia and Florida to receive the service free for a three-month period. In August of 1986 we received a subscription from our first paying client. The third partner left the company shortly thereafter. In April of 1987 we expanded the company to provide services nationwide.

Today, NurseNet has received subscriptions from more than 200 clients throughout the United States. NurseNet was designed to reduce the cost of national advertising for healthcare agencies and to serve as a centralized source of employment information for a relocating professional. Healthcare agencies do a database, we advertise in national journals, and send information to the relocating professional. The printouts include a descriptive profile of the healthcare agency, salary scale, and benefits summary. The agency receives information on all professionals who receive their printout for follow-up recruitment. Professionals seeking staff, management, or other specialized positions can use our service. We expanded our services in July, 1990, to include allied health positions.

If you really wish to start a buisness, we recommend that you get help from your local Small Business Development Center. Seek out professionals to assist you in areas of weakness, and do your research on the service or product that you will provide. Stay focused on your goals, but learn to be flexible in order to meet the needs of your customers/clients. This attribute is crucial in a service business.

Be prepared to work hard, and be willing to compromise on having a large income for a few years. If possible, try to have at least six months of personal expenses saved before starting. Remember that very few businesses have "instant success."

Remember that "no man is an island." Have a significant other in your life, whether it be a family member, spouse, or a special friend who can provide the inspiration and support that you will need when times are rough. *Always* maintain your sense of humor; you will need to be able to laugh sometimes.

If entering into a partnership, choose your partners carefully. You cannot underestimate the synergy needed to sustain a partnership. Each partner needs to recognize her/his strengths and weaknesses and utilize those strengths to achieve the overall goal of the company. There is no room in a business for insecurities or jealousies if you want your organization to succeed.

We were the first company to develop this concept of computerized referral for recruitment. Although our growth has been slower than anticipated, we know that we're on the right track because several services have evolved in the past two years attempting to simulate our concept.

If we had to leave you with one key thought, it would be: No matter what you are selling, there is always someone buying. The real questions is: do you have the energy to find them and the quality and service to turn them from prospects into customers?

If your answer to this questions is "yes," then welcome to the world of the nurse entrepreneur!

NurseNet
1422 W. Peachtree Street N.W., Suite 610
Atlanta, GA 30309
(800) 423-7568

Chapter 47

Healing the Healers

(This profile appeared in the January 1989 issue of the *Nurse Entrepreneur's Exchange*)

Editor's Note : In 1971, Sarah Stewart, CMT, CHT, CYI, was teaching vocational rehab in Hawaii when she suffered a severe head injury, subsequently resulting in seizures which required heavy medication. She went to the island of Kaui and began studying natural healing methods which included yoga, massage therapy and vegetarianism. Her seizures cleared up, and she was able to discontinue all medications.

In 1972 she became a Certified Massage Therapist, and has since taught many CMT courses. Additionally, she has developed several uniquely innovative courses for nurses, including "Healing The Healers" and "Nurturing The Nurses."

NEE: What led you to start your own practice in massage therapy?
Sarah: "In 1979, I moved to Sonoma, California, where I met a woman who did facials. I offered to trade her a massage for a facial, and was a little shaky since I hadn't given a massage for years. I did the massage and it clicked right in, and I knew I was to start doing this again. This woman was impressed, so she began referring clients as well as allowing me to use her studio as my workplace.

I still had my full-time job as a sales manager, so I only did massagestwo nights a week and on weekends. By the end of the month, I wanted to do massage full-time, so I rented a place and set up my practice. I was afraid I wouldn't be able to it financially, but I ended up being booked solid—I had as many people as I could handle.

Within six months, I'd outgrown that office, so I found a larger place and started Sarah Stewart's Body Center, which offered classes in yoga, acupuncture and rolling as well as massage therapy."

NEE: Where did the idea for your Healing the Healers class come from?
Sarah: "In 1984, I went to India by myself. And I didn't realize until I got there, and it was quiet with no phones ringing, how exhausted I was. I ate lightly, slept for days and took care of myself. That's when these visions came—if this is happening to me, how many other thousands of people who are rescuers is this happening to? And they don't even know it until they stop or until they crash and have a breakdown, or they start getting ulcers or cancers.

So that's what the focus of my work is about—we're healing the healers; we help you find tools such as hobbies, swimming, massage, yoga, and meditation that keep you from getting burned out. Taking that time to do those things for yourself—and then taking care of other people. Because you can't take care of others properly unless you are healed yourself.

I am not saying everyone has to be a vegetarian and do the same things I do. Everyone needs to find their own thing that makes them happy, but there are certain universal tools I've learned along the way that everyone can use at the time, and not wait until it's too late. Which is what most people do—they keep going and struggling and saying, 'I'll get my vacation pretty soon.' If you can take a mini-vacation every day using visualizations, meditation, taking a walk, or whatever it is that you do, then you can clear out that day's stuff without having to accumulate it over a period of time."

NEE: In 1984 you started Sarah Stewart's School of Massage to provide off-site massage certification classes.
Sarah: "Yes. In addition, I've just gotten my school approved to certify hypnotherapists and movement therapists, as well as massage therapists. I will be offering two-week certification courses in each of those areas.

I also plan to offer a six-week course that includes two weeks of massage, two weeks of hypnotherapy and two weeks of movement therapy. The students can integrate all of those forms into their work. And rather then make them separate, I'll weave them in and out during the day, which is what I do in my practice. so at the end of the six weeks, participants will be certified in all three areas."

NEE: You hold your classes at various retreat centers Why is that?
Sarah: "The only way I can do it is to take the students away from their regular environment, and have them in a place where they are taken care of where someone else cooks for them, etc. All they have to do is concentrate on studying and absorbing and healing themselves. Because during that time they will go through a personal transformation themselves.

Nutrition is a large part of it, too. In each of my retreats the diet is carefully planned. It's a diet with lots of fresh fruits, vegetables, and juices. It is a detox kind of thing, as well as helping to rebuild the body. Mostly it's to nourish the cells and increase your memory. Anyone who goes through the course comes out feeling really good and clear.

The idea is those participants then go back to Minnesota, Wisconsin, L.A., or wherever they're from, and spread the results to their clients. And after they have practiced for a time, then they too can become teachers. The idea is to empower people, not to take away their power. Most people give away their power to teachers.

Everyone has this power within them, but it has been covered up with years of old programming. Most hypnosis is dehypnosis to take out the destructive childhood programming—to clear it out and to see from your rational mind that you are clear, that you are an adult. And the clearer you get, the more you've empowered yourself to be your own healer."

NEE: Another of your retreat classes is titled Nurturing the Nurses. How did that come about?
Sarah: "Early on I got a provider number from the Board of Registered Nurses for my certification class for massage therapists, and I found that a third of my students were nurses. They would come in totally burned out and exhausted—more so than my other students. They had their own special problems and needs, so I did the first class in Hawaii in 1986.

I put it together to work with nurses to teach them how to touch other people without picking up their energy. Because doing massage, I found that if I don't shake off people's energy physically or emotionally, I'd walk around for days thinking about their problems or feeling their stuff. So I developed a way of throwing that off.

I felt that nurses needed to have that tool specifically, since they're touching people all day long and then they go home burned out. Many of them don't sleep at night, they have rotating schedules and they were starting to dread going to work. They'd have their own problems at home, and then they would go to work, and here are all these sick people to take care of with all of their stuff. Nurses often don't have a lot of time to spend with every patient, but there are certain things that you can say to that person or do for them that which allows them to be their own nurturer—so that the nurse doesn't have to do it all the time."

NEE: What effect is your work having on the healthcare system?
Sarah: "When I first started, I wanted to help liberate nurses and

doctors from hospitals! And many of my students have done that—they have started their own private practice using natural healing methods. But we don't need to leave the hospitals empty and abandon the system.

What this is doing is causing a whole transformation in the way doctors and nurses work with people. Some of the more advanced doctors are starting to grow and see that they are working with the whole person and not just the disease. The idea of nurses working under the doctor is starting to fall by the wayside because nurses are starting to empower themselves. They are the ones who are hands-on with patients all the time—they are the true healers."

Chapter 48

Making a Difference

by Mary Farrell Pawar, RN and Corrie Brouwer, RN

"We're going to start our own agency in Jersey and by this time next year be out of debt!" The four staff nurses who were in the lounge waiting to start their shift had heard me make that statement so often that they could simultaneously finish the sentence.

There were precious few certainties in that Manhattan surgical cardiac recovery unit, but there were some things you could definitely count on. If the unit was critically understaffed, there would be a transplant; if it was Christmas Eve, Dr. Bowman would do an emergency case; and if it was the beginning of a new year, they would all be hearing about my phenomenal financial future.

During the past eight years the staff had seen my business ventures run the gamut from a stint as an Amway representative to an importer/exporter whose start-up and demise were both connected to the fall of the Golden Temple in India (my husband was originally from India, thus the connection). However, during that January of 1988, I would finally start fulfilling my dream—and I would not be alone for the ride.

It was my first day off after eight 12-hour shifts in a row. I had been up since six a.m., trying to finish up those tasks one gets to only on her day off—necessary laundry, superficial cleaning, and grocery shopping.

Like many single moms, Corrie felt that she was on a constantly moving treadmill which provided very little in the way of monetary gain, no matter how hard she worked. But, on that cold January day, she had planned a day of fun and frolic. We were planning lunch together.

Leaving at noon for her one-hour drive, she emptied her mail box and started on her way. At my house, Corrie nonchalantlyl started going through her mail and noticed that her W-2 forms had arrived. She was both pleased and dismayed to find that although she had made a respectable amount of money for the year, the "bottom line" was about 50 percent less after the government had taken its share. She had no write-offs!

In order to preserve your income you need write-offs and, in order to have write-offs, you need to buy something, and, in order to buy something you need excess money, and, in order to have excess money you need to preserve your income, and, etc., etc., etc. Her decision was made, it was time for us to implement the plan we had been discussing for the previous year. On that afternoon, the consummate entrepreneur and the disgruntled tax-payer formed a partnership. What follows are some highlights of our journey.

For more than a year we had been entertaining the idea of opening a Cirtical Care Staffing Agency in New Jersey. After all, we reasoned, if such a business were headed up by two nurses who only used the most experienced and quality-conscious RNs, it could not fail. Both of us had supplemented our incomes with agency bookings in New Jersey and had seen first-hand the poor caliber of healthcare worker that many agencies were sending. We had also seen the slipshod manner in which the agencies serviced their most important clients— nurses. Well, the decision was made but now we had to figure out how to go about turning our dream into a reality.

336

Although neither of us had any formal business education, I had several resource books that covered a multitude of areas that were of interest to we two budding executives. We checked with the town where my house was located and found that the area was legally zoned for professional use. Our next call was to the county seat to find out how we could register Critical Difference, and that afternoon we paid $30.00 and formed a partnership. Of course, we first had to search the records to find out if any other business was registered under that name.

On the way back to the office (my basement!), we stopped at a local stationer, picked a logo out of a book, and ordered our stationery. The rest of the afternoon was spent on the phone with the state finding out how to get a license for the agency and how we should set up our business.

The Division of Consumer Affairs turned out to be the goverenmental agency in charge of regulating registries and temporary help firms so we spent most of our time on the phone with their office. Because we had both worked as independent contractors in the past, and felt that this was the most advantageous mode for a nurse to utilize, we applied for and obtained licensure as an Employment Agency.

It was now time to have our first board meeting, the better to make an extremely important decision—where were we going to get the money! Nurses are paid when they work a shift, hospitals take anywhere from four to six weeks to pay the agency. It would take many thousands of dollars to get started and since we had no track record, a business loan was out of the question.

That's easy, we'll work for it! Our plan was to contract ourselves through an agency in Manhattan for five to six 12-hour shifts per week and then donate the revenue from three of these shifts—each— to the fund. We reasoned that if we did this for six months, we would have roughly $50,000 to finance the business. But after a month or so, we found that working and commuting five days from five a.m. to nine a.m. was more than enough for us to handle, especially since the bulk of our shifts were done in the emergency room of a very large and somewhat unsavory inner city hospital.

For the sake of our sanity, we lowered our contributions to two shifts per week and reasoned that it would just take us a little bit longer to get the capital together.

Because we were entering a business that carried with it a number of possible liabilities, we decided that it would be wise to incorporate and thus protect ourselves from any possible personal liability. We obtained the services of a counsel and on March 1, 1988, the nurse brokerage firm of Critical Difference, Inc. was formed. We asked our attorney to draw up contracts for both the nurses and the hospitals with whom we would be doing business. But unfortunately, he was not familiar with the type of business we were conducting and we spent a great deal of money for two contract prototypes that were of no use to us in the long run.

We had learned lesson Number One in the Business School of Hard Knocks: Educate yourself before seeking the help of an expert and that way you will know for sure if s/he really is an expert!

We learned later that an attorney is not necessary to form a corporation; it can be done with a phone call to the Secretary of State and a $50.00 Incorporation Kit from a legal stationery store.

Lesson Number Two: Do not use an expensive law firm for the many mundane tasks that you can do yourself. Reserve a lawyer's services for the complex legal issues that necessitate advice of counsel.

By June, we were plugging along and banking our shifts. We had roughly $15,000. Since we were to be heading up a critical care agency, we felt that obtaining our Critical Care Registered Nurse certification was a good idea and were scheduled to take the test the following month. Of course, neither of us had any time to study so we decided to fly to Boston and take a one-day cram review with an instructor that everyone was talking about, Laura Gasparis Vonfrolio.

At that conference, two distinctive events served to launch Critical Difference into an active mode much earlier than we had anticipated. First, the head nurse of the unit we had left to do agency work—and in which we were now contracting as agency personnel and being paid twice as much—was a conference attendee. She made it quite clear that she considered us mercenaries who had jumped ship, thinking only of personal gain.

Since she had a "rule the roost" personality, she had a very hard time with two independent practitioners who were very good at their jobs and who had no need of her input. She was also incensed at the many cogent comments Laura made during the lecture about the foolishness of a nurse remaining on staff and getting half the wages of an agency person doing the same job.

The second event was meeting Laura. Her upbeat personality and encouragement served to light a fire under us and move us at a much faster rate toward our goal. "Just do it," she said. Little did we know how soon we would be taking her advice. Observing the obvious affinity that Laura felt for us only served to further alienate our former head nurse and her means of "showing us who was boss" was to refuse to book us through the agency. Since we knew that this would mean doing all of our time in that God-forsaken emergency room, we opted to get our marketing letters in the mail.

One week after taking the CCRN, I returned home to find a message on our office machine. A small north Jersey hospital wanted to meet with us in response to a letter we had sent them. An appointment was made for the next week and we were told to bring our packet with us.

Our packet—what packet? The next two days were spent utilizing a number of sources and coming up with our philosophy, several screening tests, our rates, examples of our invoice log, etc.—our packet! We hired a temp, went to a local discount store and bought a typewriter and personal copier (our first pieces of capital equipment), and spent the rest of the week having everything typed and duplicated. We bought our first business outfits, went to the meeting with the director of nurses, and walked out with our first contract! Critical Difference was now actively in business.

We used the $15,000 we had saved to support ourselves as we spent the next four weeks doing approximately 25 shifts per week. By the fifth week, our first invoice was paid and we could afford to contact two more nurses. Since we had been in nursing for such a long time, we knew a multitude of exceptional practitioners and utilized these connections. By August, our marketing letter was answered by another mid-sized hospital and we were then actively working two accounts.

By this time, we had settled down to working roughly 60 hours a week at the bedside and running the office in our "spare" time. Then, our "big break" in the staffing business came. One of the hospitals with which we had contracted was slated to launch a cardiac surgery program and had no experienced nurses to work in the recovery room. We contracted with them to supply a guaranteed number of shifts with nurse who had expertise in the field of surgical cardiac nursing.

Within six months, our business quadrupled. We were officiallly entering the big time—you could tell by the amount of debt we had acquired to finance our venture! Fortunately, our accountant was able to find us a means to finance our expansion. Within that period, two other New Jersey hospitals opened new programs and we also supplied staff for them.

In the meantime, we had moved to a "real" office building in Fairfield,

New Jersey, and added two staff members to our team who would run our office, issue checks, and book shifts. Things were steadily moving upward and it seemed that nothing could stop us.

Every few months we would talk to Laura, one of our most important mentors, and she would give us ideas or present us with opportunities. Through her, we ended up being featured in the *Wall St. Journal*.

Then, the bomb hit. We received notification from the New Jersey Department of Labor that they deemed our contractors to be employees of our company and that we were being assessed for $60,000 in unpaid employment taxes! At first we laughed, then we got angry!

The nurses with whom we contracted were well aware of their status as self-employed individuals. These were highly educated professionals who needed no direction or supervision when performing the jobs for which they had contracted. The vast majority carried private disability policies which covered them both for illness and work-related accidents that might affect their ability to work. They did not want to give up the tax advantages of filing a Schedule C and being able to deduct work-related expenses from their income. It was because of this issue that we began to meet other owners of nurse brokerage firms in our state and nationally.

Not only was the State of New Jersey interested in attacking any nurse brokerage firms who utilized independent contractors, but the Internal Revenue Service and the Department of Labor were also making it a priority to go after businesses of this type. Through the National Nursess in Business Association, a group of successful nurse-owned companies from across the nation began to meet and discuss these problems.

As a result, the Nurse Brokers and Contractors of America was formed in Washington, D.C. Critical Difference was one of the nine founding members of the group and we found ourselves among the leaders in the field. These companies were billing anywhere from five to 15 million dollars a year and several of them were on the road to going public.

Here we were again, in with the big guns. The state issue was resolved very early by a judgment in another case that went before ours. However, we spent the next two years traveling to Washington once a month to attend board meetings and try to help move the legislative issues surrounding this problem in the right direction.

Although we were unable to accomplish all the items on our agenda, NBCA has been one of the most important influences in our business. What started out as networking ended up with many wonderful and long-lasting friendships. We have gained what is probably the equivalent of a bachelor's degree in the workings of the legislative process, both local and national. Rubbing elbows with such successful entrepreneurs has definitely moved us far beyond Business 101 and has helped us to survive during very hard economic times.

Finally, we have gained the rare privilege of being able to pick up the phone at any given time and tap into the expertise of a multitude of nationally successful companies. Now that's Networking!

Just about the time that we finally got the State DOL squared away, we had to meet an even bigger obstacle, the recession at the beginning of the '90s. Staff salaries were at an all-time high, thanks to the competition from our agency, and nurses were now flocking to fill those positions because their husbands were losing their jobs. This turn of events made the need for agency work practically non-existent. Here we were, in debt up to our eyeballs so that we could support shifts that were not forthcoming.

Well, it doesn't take a genius to figure out that no shifts means no money, so we frantically started looking around for another direction. Thank goodness for supportive parents whose moral and financial support kept us going and continues to keep us afloat during the hard times.

It was another of our lunches with Laura that saved the day. For at least the fifth time, she told us that we should develop audiotapes of the Nursing State Board Review. No one was offering this review in any serious form and she thought it was a great idea. So, in January, 1992, we launched our first series, sixteen hours of lectures on audio cassette which was taped in front of a live audience.

Between January and June, we sold 800 sets nationally, and three times that amount the following year. We retape yearly in order to update and improve the series, using the evaluations sent in by students as our guide. Our instructors are student nominated and therefore represent the best of the educators nationwide. This "Circle of Excellence" is chosen from several hundred nominees each year. We now do a series for licensed practical nurses and offer audio programs which provide continuing education units for RNs. In the near future, we are planning to enter the test prep market in areas other than nursing.

Through this business, we have become educated on the logistics and mechanics of live taping, editing, and the duplication of our products. We have learned "by doing" the type of bundling and marking required to send third-class mail across the country. Currently, we reach our market through a national mailing to 225,000 students and by advertising in several national nursing journals. We do on-site presentations at local and national student conventions and provide incentives for students to represent us at the conventions we cannot attend. However, our best advertisements are student-to-student recommendations. After tracking our advertising to measure its effectiveness, we found that referral doubled the first year and quadrupled the second and third years.

We became particularly interested in the audio-learning field after utilizing the business and motivational programs of Nightingale Conant, a multi-million dollar business and unchallenged leader in the audio education field. We plan to become the Nightingale Conant of Nursing!

Because we take the time to edit our tapes and choose educators whose style and content are unsurpassed, we believe that no other company will measure up to our product. We know that students prefer to listen to our lively and informative lectures at their own convenience and as often as they wish. It is our belief in our product, our willingness to work as long and as hard as is necessary, and our downright ornery persistence that helped us actualize our goals.

Critical Difference, Inc.
Advantage Healthcare
12 East Drive
Stanhope, NJ 07874
Mary Pawar, Cory Brouwer
201-573-8995   Fax 201-882-6995

Chapter 49

NNBA:
An Inside Look

(This profile appeared in the May 1990 issue of the Nurse-Entrepreneur's Exchange.)

Editor's Note: The National Nurses in Business Association (NNBA), two years old this May, is currently the only existing national organization dedicated to promoting independent nursing practice through the entrepreneurial model.

Of NNBA's 500+ nationwide members, approximately 50 percent own and operate a healthcare-related business; the other half are exploring entrepreneurial or alternative healthcare career options.

On this, NNBA's second anniversary, we interviewed David Norris, RN, NNBA's founder and executive director, to provide a closer look at this unique organization.

NEE: What events led you to start NNBA?

David: "By 1985, I had been a hospital nurse for thirteen years, and was beginning to burn out. Patient care was still rewarding, but I was weary of unsatisfying clinical practice environments due to institutional politics and ineffective management policy. It was the classic "I love my work but I hate my job' syndrome.

After reading the book Nurses in Business by Margo Neal, I was convinced entrepreneurship provided the most effective way to control one's practice environment, so I conducted a literature search on nurse entrepreneurs—and found practically nothing!

So I began publishing the Nurse-Entrepreneur's Exchange, the forerunner of this newsletter. By 1987, subscribers were asking for more information and networking support than could be included in the newsletter, so I began to explore the idea of expanding into a national organization.

Since I didn't have the money to hire a staff, I was reluctant to attempt the undertaking on my own. Knowing how much work it would entail, I was afraid it would simply be overwhelming, considering I would still have to support myself through ICU nursing for an indeterminate time. I waited around for months, hoping someone else would do it first! No one did, and it seemed to be a natural evolution of my efforts—so in May of 1988 I jumped in with both feet."

NEE: Why did you take the unusual step of structuring NNBA as a for-profit organization?

David: "Our purpose is to foster independent nursing practice, primarily through entrepreneurship, but also intrapreneurship as well. In a nutshell, our philosophy is that the root cause of the nursing crisis is the dependent nature of nursing practice. Because of the lack of autonomy, nurses are not perceived as professionals. This perception has resulted in the dramatic decline of people choosing nursing as a career. Last year, more women applied to medical school than to nursing school? Why? Because becoming a physician means prestige, power, and money—everything traditional nursing lacks. This is the recruitment aspect of the nursing shortage.

The other factor in the shortage is retention. While studies show that most nurses are working as nurses, I believe that the number of nurses dissatisfied with the traditional practice environment is increasing. I think we're

346

on the verge of a mass exodus of nurses from the field unless nursing practice is reorganized.

Many nurses, myself included, believe that the collective solution is for nurses to create corporations that contract nursing services to facilities. These nurses will be independent contractors, not employees. Facilities would be relieved of staffing and personnel-associated costs and responsibilities, and the corporate nurses would enjoy autonomy, respect, and higher salaries. They would also be more accountable—something most nurses and their patients desire. Individually, nurses are increasingly starting their own healthcare businesses; the variety of services offered by our members is inspiring."

NEE: What effect has NNBA had on you personally and professionally?

David: "I've experienced the personal satisfaction of taking an idea from concept to reality. I have attained the goal of being my own boss—I resigned my hospital job in February of 1989, and have been directing NNBA full-time since then. So far, I have earned less than a staff nurse salary, and that situation definitely needs to improve, but NNBA has been in the black since day one. Im' quite pleased about that.

Professionally, I have the pleasure of associating with the most dynamic group of nurses imaginable. Entrepreneurs by nature are gutsy individualists, who, not content with the status quo, change it to suit their dreams and needs. Our members have done exactly that, and in doing so are speeding nursing's evolution by expanding its frontiers. They give me hope for the future of nursing. And I am blessed with the charge of spreading the word of their work and achievements, which in turn helps others to do the same. What better kind of work could I ask for?"

NEE: What are some current NNBA activities?

David: "We've just completed creating our first Executive Advisory Board, who will be giving valuable input into the direction of the association. We are also developing Regional Coordinator guidelines, in order to set up regional chapters across the country. And, of course, our second annual conference is this month. I'm thrilled with the variety of sessions planned, and expect we'll reach our goal of 500 attendees. Our keynote speaker this year, Venner Farley, EdD, RN, is one of the most dynamic public speakers I've ever heard. Last year, at our first annual conference, many attendees said that it was the most exciting conference they had ever attended—that's a reputation I hope will become a tradition for all NNBA conferences."

NEE: What about NNBA's future?

David: "NNBA is a young, grassrotts organization that promises to grow along with the movement it represents. Most entrepreneurial-minded nurses still have never heard of us. They are a tough group to reach because they are not easily identifiable. Word-of-mouth referrals are increasing, and that helps a lot. I'm also having articles and press releases published with increasing frequency — that, of course, helps too.

My vision is to see NNBA develop and implement a pilot project that would establish an independent nursing corporation that contracts to provide nursing services to an entire hospital. I'm confident this project would prove to be successful. It could thus serve as model for similar projects nationwide. NNBA is uniquely positioned, and has the human resources among our members to accomplish it."

National Nurses in Business Association
56 McArthur Avenue
Staten Island, NY 10312
(800) 331-6534
FAX# 718-317-0858

Chapter 50

Getting Started...

by Glenna B. Mills, BSN, and Katherine T. Pollin, MBA, BSN

For a few moments, we pore over travel brochures, avidly savoring the descriptions of idyllic resorts. We feel the bright tropical sun tempered by warm sea breezes; we hear the crunching of the sand under our feet and the plaintive cry of the sea birds looking for a meal over the ocean's edge.

It takes a little while to feel the impact of reality: the bright sun is the desk light, the warm sea breeze is provided by a small desk fan, the crunching sand is the soft insistence of the phone, and the plaintive cry of the sea birds is really the office cat meowing reproachfully that, while he admires our dedication to hard work and long hours, he would really appreciate being fed on schedule—if it is not too much trouble.

We enjoyed the vacation vicariously, but real vacations will have to wait. There is work to be done!

We started our corporation because we wanted the challenge and stimulation of applying our skills and experience to our own business. As professional colleagues with many years experience in home healthcare, we knew we could provide a desired and valued service to California home healthcare providers.

Over many long dinners, cups of coffee, and numerous telephone conversations, we built a service organization on paper. *Plan,plan,plan* became the guiding words for several months. We talked to colleagues, investigated the market, the competition, and the opportunities. We chose an accountant and an attorney, and we listened, evaluated, and made our decisions carefully. Our respective families supported our efforts as they ran errands, input data into the computer, and freely offered advice. We read books and more books. (We even took a book to our attorney to share with her.) Workshops offered by SCORE, the IRS, and other organizations gave us new insights into our business venture.

We educated our consultants about nursing and home healthcare, and bit by bit designed a management consultation service which would cover all facets of the home health industry. We would offer "turnkey" agency start-up or "guidance-only" services for do-it-yourself advocates.

The development process inevitably led us to design home healthcare and business developmment classes for continuing education credit. These classes rapidly became an integral part of our business.

We decided upon a professional corporation as our legal form of business, and the incorporation process loomed over us as a monster—a blur of do, don't, and why not? We talked to people, asked questions, and developed a plan. We selected our attorney because she was experienced in corporate law, highly recommended, and because she was willing to guide us as we did most of the work. We presented her with a well conceived outline of our organization and became versed in the process of incorporation. In reality, incorporating turned out to be as easy as "rolling off a log," and the careful preparation saved us many dollars. Finally, Mills, Pollin & Associates, Inc., A Professional Nursing Corporation was a reality!

We searched for the "best buy" in liability insurance for the corporation: the quotes ranged from $2,500 per year to $25,000 per year (obviously, that firm wasn't interested in our business). It seemed they wanted to peg us as providers of home care services, and it was finally through networking that we found affordable coverage.

It seems hard to believe that choosing color, style, and format for the letterhead would be more time consuming and difficult then actually putting our work on paper! We thoughtfully chose the blend of color, style, and format that would become our trademark, be a reflection of our business, and project an image of ourselves.
Being aware of the reefs and shoals ahead made deciding on a home office relatively easy. We checked out the benefits of a home office, waded through contradictory legal and accounting advice, made our decision, and another hurdle was behind us. We would not have clients visiting our office, so a home office was cost-effective and very convenient. But working at home poses some challenges, too; you need to pretend that you are going to a *real* office, ignore the "home work" (and the refrigerator), and concentrate on the work ahead!

Typical of most small businesses, we funded our enterprises personally. As a corporation, we each bought 50 percent of the shares, which provided us with the money we required for start-up operation. Our stock certificates were admired and then safely tucked away in our individual safe deposit boxes.

Now we are incorporated (since 1989), have our stationery, our new computer, telephone line and 800 number, and money (a modest amount, to be sure, but it was there as corporate funds). This was not a time to relax, but a time to unleash the power of entrepreneurship, to go forth and succeed!

Our first contract came shortly after our opening. Celebration was in order and then more celebration when our first check arrived. The check was promptly photocopied, admired by our families, and reverently deposited. The photocopy was appropriately framed and hung on the wall in a place of honor. After months of planning, we were in business.

Eager to continue our successful start-up, we continued our marketing efforts with enthusiasm. We renewed old acquaintances and developed new contacts, wrote letters, and made follow-up calls, constantly developing an ever-expanding circle of potential clients. Advertisements for our consulting services and continuing education classes appeared in trade magazines and nursing journals. We developed brochures, stuffed envelopes with the assistance of ever-willing family members, learned about mass mailings, and conquered the whims of the postage meter.

Our first experience as exhibitors at a home healthcare conference was fun, instructive, and exhausting! Most of all, it was rewarding. We had developed a new product line, a computerized version of a policy manual, to introduce at this meeting. This sparked immediate interest among health agency administrators and gave birth to new contracts.

One cannot rest on her laurels; as we work with clients today, we market for clients tomorrow. We stay constantly on our toes (tiring, but necessary) as we evaluate our services, keep abreast of the changing home healthcare environment, and adjust accordingly.

We think of the present and the future simultaneously. Our learning will never cease; we must constantly hone our current skills and learn new ones, cherish old values, but open our minds to new ideas.

The rewards come in many forms. It is great to have the opportunity to help others achieve their goals, to use our collective knowledge and experience to meet new challenges, and to take responsibility and credit for our corporate success!

Mills, Pollin & Associates, Inc.
A Professional Nursing Corporation
1921 Augustus Court
Walnut Creek, CA 94598
(415) 937-7563
(800) 728-4817